THAT HEALING FEELING

The Convergence of Faith and Medicine

Jean A. Pentico

THAT HEALING FEELING
The Convergence of Faith and Medicine

The Rhodes-Fulbright Library

by Jean A. Pentico

ProdCode: CSS/250/361/4.48/24

Library of Congress
Catalog in Publication

00-11248

International Standard Book Number

1-55605-321-5

Printed in the United States of America

Wyndham Hall Press
Bristol, IN   46507-9460

TO

DR. BERNIE S. SIEGEL WHOSE WORDS ENCOURAGED ME
WHEN FEW PEOPLE KNEW WHAT I WAS EXPERIENCING,
LEARNING OR PRACTICING

In memory of Lucy

A special thanks to Dr. James Kalar whose medical expertise
includes an open mind, wisdom, intuition and trust.

CONTENTS

INTRODUCTION

My hospital roommate's cancer had spread throughout her body. Her doctors didn't know what was keeping her alive. Repeatedly I watched and heard her religious rituals. It was obvious when she felt revitalized because her audible prayers were those of thanksgiving and praise. I could have told the doctors why she was surviving. I had been doing the same thing for several years.

That was at the beginning of my forty-year journey with "healing feelings". However, it wasn't long before I realized nothing new had entered my body. The healing chemistry was already there! It was evident that specific religious emotions were stimulating healing mechanisms. THAT HEALING FEELING explains how I learned to consciously develop and use these sensations in a biofeedback manner.

Recent medical science abounds with research supporting the vital role emotions play in health, healing and the creation of life. In THAT HEALING FEELING information is correlated which approaches the subject of faith healings from a view most Christians may not have considered. The gift of healing is already ours. We can learn to employ these healing mechanisms in our bodies.

Drs. Herbert Benson, Bernie Siegel, Deepak Chopra, Andrew Weil and many more have emphasized the power the mind has over the body. For years this has been one of the most popular subjects in the media.

We now know more at the molecular level. From the vital role of emotions in creating cells of life, to the recognition of belief systems capable of spontaneously changing the DNA of cells, the mysteries are becoming realities.

When I first knew what it was like to be healed through faith, I was convinced of its reality. What I experienced was real and of the real world.

Once I started this writing, the scientific and logical data supporting my perspective began emerging from numerous sources. I could not have imagined such a horde of useful information would be unfolding around me.

I write not because I have experienced something unique. On the contrary what has happened to me has occurred in some relative form to countless people throughout the centuries of religious history. Faith healings have been described many times throughout Christianity. This includes a significant number in the Bible.

I did not know if I could explain the body processes and chemical changes brought about through faith but I knew I could begin with what I did understand. I could explain what has worked for me. At the same time I could attempt to pull together factual information which was comprehensible.

This did not mean God was not the source of healing. It did not mean God was excluded from the picture. If I was convinced healings were of the world of reality, I was also convinced God was real.

The main focus of this writing is to emphasize how important an individual's faith, thoughts, emotions and beliefs can be in healing. My deepest conviction is that no one, when faced with a health crisis, needs to assume there is nothing they can do beyond medical help. I am convinced that medical help augments the incredible life forces present in our body mechanisms. As individuals we can enhance all healing processes with our minds.

As I write, my understandings evolve. It is fitting that they do so. This is hallowed ground. It is appropriate that understandings on this subject should evolve in keeping with the patterns of the universe.

CHAPTER I

THE LIFE FORCE

"I maintain that cosmic religious feeling is the strongest and noblest incitement to scientific research."

Albert Einstein

What is the essence of life? What is the human "spirit"? When a person is in a hospital intensive-care unit and is hooked to machines that keep them breathing, their heart beating and their kidneys functioning, what is it that makes the difference between life and death? Doctors usually recommend disconnecting life support systems when the brain signals have stopped as indicated by an electroencephalogram or EEG. At this point people appear to be brain dead. The spirit or soul, some believe, is no longer there.

It is in this narrow borderline between life and death that people have often recalled white light experiences or mysterious encounters with someone from heaven. We each interpret these kinds of experiences according to our perspectives and beliefs.

It is one thing to view them from the outside looking in and it is another to consider them as the participator. I had an encounter that could fall into this category without some of the ramifications others have described. For days my fever had ranged well over one hundred and four degrees (104°). As I lay in a hospital bed I felt surrounded by a bright white light. My weakness was overwhelming. I couldn't lift my eyelids.

My husband had just asked how I was feeling. As I was struggling to say the words that would describe my feelings, the doctor arrived. My husband explained my weakness to him.

Immediately the doctor roughly lifted my eyelids and flashed a light into them. He was not at all gentle, as other doctors had been.

I became angry. Suddenly I felt energy surge within my body and my extreme weakness became noticeably improved.

Years later, in retrospect, I recognized that it was a surge of adrenalin as the result of my anger that brought me back from the brink of death. This became my first awareness of the vital force of emotions in life.

It was emotion that made the difference between life and death for me. In that instance emotion was my life force. This opened whole vistas of emotion. I couldn't help but wonder how they were involved in making up the life force.

Today scientific understandings tell us all thoughts are emotionally interpreted in the brain. Thoughts alone could account for a myriad of interpretations but in order to consider this question we need to look at the broader view. There are more than thoughts being emotionally interpreted. Sights, sounds, smells, external and internal physical sensations are constantly being evaluated with some kind of emotion. This is done relative to whether these sensations enhance or diminish life in its struggle to survive.

Just as there are many relative forms of life happenings to emotionally interpret, there are numerous kinds of these feelings that constantly occur. We are only aware of those emotions that come to our conscious awareness.

All of these interactions in the brain draw upon past similar events for comparison. With vast amounts of experiences recorded, the activity of each translation is greatly multiplied. We begin to see a picture of the brain with millions of interactions as all thoughts and sensations are evaluated relative to ongoing experiences. With each translation the brain produces chemicals that direct the body in its needs for life. Due to nueropeptides much of this is done within moments.

Because of emotional interactions, the life force is created. These vast interpretations call for things like the production of adrenalin, thyroid, estrogen, endorphins and much more. With built-in controls, life creates its own energy- -its life force.

Suddenly the role of emotions is turned upside down. Past emotions could get in the way of logic and reason. Emotions were the frosting on the cake of life but not the nuts and bolts of human existence.

Emotions, in fact, are closely related to our sensuousness and therefore they are involved in religious concepts of sin and evil doings. Often emotions have not been a favorite component of life for they are involved in hysteria, frenzy and uncontrolled behavior.

For decades many studies have been done which demonstrate that negative emotions such as stress, tension, anxiety and anger are included in the picture of the development of disease. Everything from tooth decay to heart disease and cancer have been related to these negative feelings.

For more than forty years the influences of negative emotions have made medical news. Positive feelings have just begun to take their rightful place in their contribution to health and survival.

It should be noted that when a person is unconscious or asleep, automatic mechanisms take over. During sleep, regular periods of dreams occur drawing upon past emotional events and experiences. When a person is seriously ill, the events can become more dramatic such as delirium or hallucinations. Always there is a purpose and reason.

Once, when I was delirious, I experienced a musical marching band as it crossed my chest. Another time an awesomely brilliant blue butterfly was seen. These were not ordinary experiences. Why? Because my body was calling for extraordinary chemistry to bring me back to wellness.

The white light experience could easily fall into these kinds of built-in life forces or survival reactions. The near death white light experience is ethereal, heavenly. The feelings encountered at that time are outstanding, life-giving ones, relative to the body's needs.

Life always struggles to survive. In life is the Supreme Wisdom of creation.

For over six billion years the universe has been evolving honing, perfecting and correcting itself. The mere fact that we are alive in this part of the twentieth century implies that incredible honing and perfecting processes have preceded us through eons of time. It implies that there is far more "good" in our humanness than we have begun to comprehend. Emotions are part of that goodness.

All emotions call for the production of body chemicals. These chemicals produce the energy that makes up the life force for each of us. A spirit is a name we have always given to an energy or force we couldn't understand. It now appears that our emotional life force is synonymous with our spirit.

"Is that all there is?" In the words of a popular song from the fifties, is that all there is to the human spirit?

It would be a mistake to ignore the fact that it was a thought that preceded that life saving surge of adrenalin for me years ago. The thought came from me, my mind, my brain. It was the result of my personality. Someone else might have seen the rough eyelid treatment as another reason to give up. Another person might have ignored the bodily insult entirely. My personality responded the way it did because of who I am.

Personalities are made up of countless experiences, our emotional interpretations of them and our intellectual responses in each instance. This is why we are unique individuals.

Because of my personality, a thought was formed that led to my feelings of anger. It is true that without the thought there would have been no surge of adrenalin. Still the thought, itself, did not create the energy. It was the emotional interpretation that caused the surge of adrenalin that brought me back from the edge of death.

The fact remains that I am something beyond my emotional energy. Yet without that energy is there a life force? Can I exist without a life force? And how does the human will fit into the picture of spirit and personality? Human will is sometimes given credit for survival. Some people are said to be strong willed.

Then there is the question of what leaves the body when we die? In religion what do we believe goes to heaven when we die? So far we have not mentioned the word, soul. Is the soul the same as our life force, personality or spirit? There are well known psychiatrists who insist the soul is our mind. By contrast there are many famous Christian hymns that proclaim religious feelings are experienced down in one's soul. This implies it is part of one's body. Often it is described as somewhere in the chest or near the solar plexus. What is it, then, that leaves the body at the time of our death?

Perhaps it is best described as the essence of life. Perhaps who we are and what we've done, what we have accomplished and how we have handled our lives is part of the total picture of that which lives on beyond us. If this is the case, each life is important to all whose lives they have touched. Each is held in high esteem or looked down upon depending upon their deeds. There are famous people who have influenced other lives in positive ways for centuries through their art, music, scientific discoveries, literature and more. Our loved ones live on in our thoughts, memories and influences.

For some people these concepts of life after death are enough. It should come as no surprise, then, that some Christians and pastors have been focusing on such aspects of life after death for years.

There are concepts of streets paved with gold, descriptions of thrones and angels singing night and day. There are many teachings about life after death. It would hardly be appropriate to take all of them literally. We need to periodically reevaluate our religious beliefs in the mystical in light of logic and the latest scientific understandings about creation.

CHAPTER II

FAITH HEALINGS

"We need to reimagine what we think we understand."

...Thomas Moore

Mention the term "faith healing" and medical people rapidly divide into two groups. There are those who have seen healings or spontaneous remissions for which they have no logical answer. There is another group, perhaps the larger one, who assumes the illness was misdiagnosed in the first place or the illness must have been psychosomatic. Therefore, there truly was no healing when the person felt well again.

Often spontaneous remissions are viewed as something unrelated to faith healings. Because the hallowed ground of religious occurrences restricts understandings, research is limited. Still, if the mechanisms exist for spontaneous remissions, it is quite logical that they are a relative form of the mechanisms that are at work in faith healings. And while spontaneous remissions are rare, Drs. Elmer and Alice Green at Menninger's Clinic studied an impressive number of four hundred cases.

It is a strange dichotomy that in our highly advanced society where mysticism is taken out of reproduction, digestion, respiration and countless other biological functions, the disease reversal phenomenon remains mysterious.

It is much easier to forget that digestion, reproduction and even the cause of bacterial diseases were all considered to be acts of God at one time. The fact that a gradual understanding of some of these processes evolved over centuries explains our present day casual attitude regarding them. As awesome as they remain, the mysteries of these biological functions are largely understood. As the result, such processes are no longer viewed as they were many centuries ago.

What is most surprising, however, is the fact that medical science, with its vast knowledge today, has crossed the bridge to understanding faith healings. This has been done, for the most part, without their awareness. It is information that has been gleaned for other reasons and from a variety of sources.

There are broad Christian views on the subject of faith healings. Certainly the vast majority of us believe in medical help when we are ill.

Modern "miracles" of medicine such as heart and liver transplants place us in awe of such accomplishments.

Yet our Christian tradition, based upon Biblical teachings, emphasizes the reality of faith healings. Whole branches of Christianity have continued this emphasis. Christian Science churches teach healings through faith. Every year thousands of people journey to Catholic shrines seeking healings.

I grew up knowing wonderful Pentecostal families who rejected medical science and trusted God to heal them when they were sick. Faith healings have been a strong tradition within Christianity throughout the years.

This has not been without tragedies. There have been failed healings that caused broken bones or other serious repercussions. There have been charlatan practitioners and fraudulent demonstrators. Much pain and suffering has resulted from these kinds of practices that could hardly be considered the ideal.

It is logical and important that better connections be made between medical science and religious healings.

In the sixties I shared a hospital room with a young woman who had cancer. Her nurse confided in me that her cancer had spread throughout her body. Her doctors, I was told, did not know what was keeping her alive. Over and over I watched and heard and saw her petition God in prayer and adoration. It was always obvious when she felt revitalized because she switched to prayers of appreciation and thankfulness. This was followed by more adoration.

I could have told the doctors why she was surviving. I had been doing the same thing for several years.

In the beginning I had relied upon the same kinds of religious rituals my hospital roommate used. In time, however, I realized nothing new had entered my body. There were new sensations as the result of strong convictions but no new healing chemistry had suddenly entered my body. I was convinced the chemistry and the pathways were already there. It was *religious feelings* that had amplified my healing body chemistry.

From the beginning there were some things I was sure of. The rate of speed with which the energizing occurred was faster than that of chemicals or hormones circulating through the blood. I could relate it to thoughts of anger or fear where there is an instantaneous response. It seemed to be a nerve reaction, because of its speed, but the mechanisms for such things were only partially known then.

I did know what I had experienced and I began to analyze the feelings: where, how and what I felt. In time I learned to consciously imitate them. Convinced that I couldn't be the only one in the world with these understandings, I searched other ancient religions for evidence of sensations that were used in energizing or healing exercises. Most of them had their roots in the Far East but they did exist. They were meditation exercises.

I developed mind-body techniques which fall into the category of biofeedback exercises today. I have used these exercises for decades to reverse many things from breast lumps to carpal tunnel pain, leg cramps and more. Sometimes it was months before I learned a workable technique. For instance by concentrating on my carpal tunnel pain I made it worse in the beginning. By contrast I can get relief in a minute or two today. Each new health problem requires reevaluation. When I want the best results, I always go back to the original religious exercises.

It should be noted that my hospital roommate, Laura, had healings that lasted for short periods of time. Some of mine have been like that, too. Although the energizing happens within minutes, the effects last for a few hours.

Although it may sound discouraging to need to repeat religious exercises ever few hours, it could never be described as unpleasant or uncomfortable. On the contrary they are always uplifting experiences with great rewards.

A person could rationalize that most medications are taken every few hours. Therefore these healing exercises could be compared to medicine.

There have been advantages to these short healing episodes. In the process, the mystery has been diminished while the reality of the process has increased.

While I have one health problem that has returned numerous times, other healings are permanent. One happened not long ago. We had just acquired a new dog whose enthusiasm needed to be curbed. In order to restrict his activities, I blocked the steps going upstairs with clothes hampers and other tall containers.

Our main living area is the lower level of a split entry home where the floor is cement.

Coming down the steps I got caught as I was attempting to go over the barricade. Awkwardly I landed with my full two hundred pounds on my sixty five-year-old knees.

As I lay moaning and groaning on the floor, I suddenly had the sense to switch to the concentration of healing energy for my knees. In a few minutes I was able to painlessly walk. Furthermore, I had no unpleasant repercussions the next day. Except for a small black and blue area on the side of my one knee, there were no further problems.

A skeptic would say that nothing could be proved in an episode like this. Maybe my knees weren't damaged. Maybe I wouldn't have had problems anyway.

I know these healings work because they have helped me countless times for more than thirty years. I cannot pretend to understand all facets of all kinds of faith healings. My concern is that the kind I do understand are likely to be the most common kind. However, how many people know that a single success that later fails can be regained through the same steps of faith, prayer and adoration? That repeating this over and over again may be quite necessary? How many people know that they need to get involved with feelings of adoration, awe and love? That waiting for someone else or God to do something for them is not the only answer?

THAT HEALING FEELING

Faith healings come from God, it's true.
But there's one step we need to do.
Our body chemistry is changed,
Disease and healing rearranged,
By what we think and what we feel- -
And praising God can make it real!
It's more than just a mental thought
That brings the healing we have sought.
It's adoration, awe and love,
And feeling all of the above.
This heals our souls and bodies too,
And that's the step that we can do.
Christ emphasized our vital role
When He said faith can make you whole.
Christ made it clear when He would say
Your faith has made you whole today.

Jean A. Pentico

CHAPTER III

WHOLENESS

When we say we feel well, what do we really mean? In an era of laser perfection, computers and space travel, our language often seems inadequate. At first, feeling well seems to imply feeling physically well. But we know it really means much more.

We are also feeling positive emotionally. We may be feeling happy, enthusiastic, loving, eager, energetic, jovial, etc.

The ancients had a term for feeling well. It was called feeling whole. If a person was sick they were not whole. Biblical accounts of healings are often stated as feeling whole or being made whole.

Today, thousands of years later, we can understand what they meant. We have come full circle. We know the mind cannot be separated from the body and emotions. They are all integrated into one whole. When we have happy thoughts, within an instant our body feels happy. When we become angry the body responds in a flash.

The concept of the mind's relationship to the body's health has been an uncomfortable one from the beginning of scientific research.

It was bad enough when the Bible made statements that insisted people's sin caused their disease. In the Biblical era people even believed the blindness of a child could be blamed on the sins of a parent. Guilt was being thrown around left and right.

It appeared that medical research was doing the same thing with their concepts of stress, anxiety and disease. We were forced to consider that we played a vital role in the development of our own disease. Although this principle caused people to feel some guilt about their behavior, it was usually rationalized away, even though scientific studies supported these discoveries.

Besides, there were serious illnesses like cancer that caused much pain and suffering. Who wanted to add guilt to the suffering of these people and their families? What about sweet Aunt Matilda who died of breast cancer? Or dear Mother Tillie who died of bone cancer? Death hardly seemed like something a person could take lightly or place in the realm of thought control.

If feeling good and feeling well translate into a rainbow of positive emotions that produce the proper chemistries for wellness, one can't help but wonder if a person can feel "good" and be sick. Obviously, where cancer is concerned, people often feel good for a long time before their disease is discovered. And on the other end of the spectrum, we all know people who are happy and cheerful in spite of a serious or even fatal illness.

A common question in this whole scenario of mind-body health is why don't these positive thinkers who are happy and cheerful, in spite of their fatal disease, get well? Why do happy, patient, courageous, devout, religious people die?

Clearly, we are all going to die sometime so that isn't the question. Having said that, the next question is whether these people could influence their own wellness and recovery?

Growing trends in wholistic medicine indicate they can. Mental imagery, relaxation techniques, support groups and getting in touch with one's true feelings are some of the positive approaches.

There is strong evidence for the relationship between feelings and disease reversals. In every case of spontaneous remissions studied by the Greens at Menningers there had been a change in attitude, perspectives, thoughts and feelings that preceded their remissions.

It is a common portion of wholistic medicine to be real, know yourself, deal with hidden fears, angers and pain. This encourages spontaneous emotions that have also been shown to be more successful in disease reversals.

A lot has been said about emotions. We were created with an emotional capacity for a reason. Anger and fear were essential for survival in the processes of evolution. Love and the pleasurable feelings of sex have been necessary for the survival of the species. Some of these feelings are known to cause more serious problems than desired.

And, yes, there are emotional feelings that are not conducive to healings. From my experience crying as a brief respite during tension can relieve stress. But a lengthy pity party can make a person feel worse when they are trying to get well. Extended worry, anger, sorrow, fear, and self-pity can be destructive.

If the ancients made the profound point that wholeness is wellness, the Bible also clearly states that it is your faith that makes you whole or well. Christ especially emphasized this vital role when he said over and over again that it is your faith that makes you whole.

Why? Faith involves religious thoughts. Faith changes fear, anger and worry. Emotional interpretations of religious thoughts affect the body. Although dynamic, dramatic healings are known to occur, it is the less obvious ones that we need to recognize. They have been misunderstood and ignored.

Since neither Laura nor I had permanent healings we needed to repeat these concentration exercises every few hours. It should be noted that although the healing energy, the feelings of wellness, were instantaneous they usually needed to be performed many times in succession to achieve the few hours of wellness we enjoyed each time. Laura's prayers would often last twenty minutes. I have sometimes spent an hour in meditation, depending upon the seriousness of the situation.

There are a number of things that influence the length of time needed for feeling "well". One is the seriousness of the health problem, as I just mentioned. Another influencing factor is whether the problem is life threatening or relates to a specific area or location in the body.

I also think the length of time the health problem has existed may have some bearing on the results. For instance my recent recovery from the knee injuries took place in a matter of minutes, probably due to the fact that very little time had lapsed before I shifted to the healing concentration.

I can also attest to the fact that experience makes a difference. Learning to influence my carpal tunnel problems took time to work out, but once I learned what to do, the results were rapid and successful. Considering I was about to lose the strength in my hands some years ago, I am thankful.

Another factor involved in healings is one's personality, their faith and beliefs. Perseverance, patience and determination are obviously helpful, too. However, it is a mistake to put restrictions on healing possibilities. Since neither Laura nor I had achieved permanent healings they seem to be in a separate category. Yet logic would suggest that it is far more likely the same mechanisms are at work but there is something else involved.

It could be related to the kinds of past surgeries a person has experienced and the body hormones that are no longer naturally produced. While things like thyroid and estrogen can be successfully replaced by medication, they are not available to be spontaneously manufactured, as they may be needed for a healing.

People experience feelings differently. They internalize them on varying levels. Perhaps people who have permanent healings have religious feelings on deeper levels. This breaks through to chemistry that completes the healing.

Psychosomatic illnesses seem to be an integral part of this whole mind-body picture of health. If the mind can make the body physically sick, can the mind make the body physically well? If, through religious emotional exercises, the body can be made to feel well often enough, can a person overcome an otherwise serious disease by allowing the body to heal itself?

There are some rigid medical guidelines for healings which some branches of Christianity follow before they claim a healing as a miracle. What if the medical guidelines have been incorrect? What if religious people have been mistaken?

I am convinced there are far more minor healings that (a) people don't talk about because they don't want to sound weird, (b) someone didn't realize their worshipful emotions played a major role in their feeling well, and (c) some sudden unexplainable change in a patient's condition caused the illness to be classified as psychosomatic by a doctor.

An example comes to mind regarding an older lady who shared a hospital room with me years ago. I was awakened at sunrise to sounds of prayer and emotion coming from behind her bed curtain. When her doctor arrived at 7:00 a.m., he commented on how much better she looked than he had seen in a long time.

It is apparent to me now why she looked better. What is also apparent is that if she had repeated those religious rituals at 10:00 a.m. she probably would have looked and felt better again.

Emotions and women have a long history. This has not always been pleasant. However, for years men have been said to have more heart attacks because they are more likely to bottle up their stress and tension. In the mean time women have been living longer and their emotional honesty has been getting much of the credit. Ironically, in recent decades as women have taken on the responsibility of more male oriented roles in the business world, heart attacks and other male stress-related illnesses have increased in women.

Throughout the centuries as specific branches of Christianity evolved that placed a major emphasis on faith healings, they often denounced medical help. There is a certain logic in this. One hundred per cent belief in something or someone is much more effective than partial belief. Even doctors know that medicine can fail if patients don't believe in their treatment or medicine.

I have a great deal of confidence in medical doctors. They helped save my life when my appendix burst and twice when I had peritonitis. I'd much rather have a good antibiotic for a serious sore throat than try to heal it through concentration. I take thyroid and estrogen medications which I would not want to be without at this point in my life.

The whole issue is not one of faith healings or medicine. The problem is one of understandings so that the best of two worlds can be combined for the greatest benefit to people who are in need.

There is another aspect of wholeness. It is often described as feeling at one with God. It is a oneness with the perfection, wisdom, beauty and power of creation- -all that has preceded us in our existence; all that surrounds and supports us in our life.

How can that be? Some experts agree that all steps of our evolving life are recorded in our brains. Certainly the information in our DNA evolved eons ago. We are consciously aware of a minute portion of who we really are. In a religious experience it is possible that we get in touch with the greater Whole. Perhaps processes in our brain interact with those forces in our bodies that have contributed to our wholeness and they merge as one awesome experience.

There are hints as to how this could happen. When I first realized no new chemistry had entered my body in a healing experience and I looked for other relative forms, I had a puzzling episode. I had gone to a chiropractor regarding a back problem. As he was manipulating the back of my spine and approached the base of my neck, a feeling of euphoria swept over me. This was puzzling because I certainly had no thought that was grand enough to cause such a sensation. Neither did anything physical feel that good. While I would not describe euphoria the same as a religious experience, it would fall into the category of relative forms because of its dynamics and wondrous feelings.

In the rapidly growing field of neurobiology it is recognized that the hypothalamus acts as the head of the autonomic nerves and endocrine system and provides the substructure of emotional behavior and psychic experience. Neurotransmitters and neuropeptides act upon the hypothalamus, which is at the base of the brain.

In other words the manipulation of my back up the spine could have released unusual amounts of neuropeptides which acted upon the hypothalamus causing the feelings of euphoria. Religious feelings are not unrelated to this phenomenon.

THE SECOND COMING

Precision in every atom!
Intelligence in ever cell!
Why do we believe God is real?
Can't you see? Don't you know? Can't you tell?

Why do we worship our Maker?
Why do we adore Him and sing?
He is the Lord of Creation
He is in, of and with all things.

Coming from high holy places,
Descending from heaven above,
He is the center of being.
He's the source of all life and love.

Looking in all the wrong places?
Denying that He could exist?
The seed has already been planted.
Look inside yourself, lest He be missed.

Jean A. Pentico

CHAPTER IV

THE PLEASURE PRINCIPLE

From the beginnings of all life forms, what "feels good" has been life promoting. From simple celled plants that reach for the sun, to birds that fly south for the winter, to humans who surround themselves with pleasurable things, good feelings have been life promoting. The reactions are primitive. They are essential. Mechanisms of some kind that are capable of registering and conveying such messages exist in all living things.

Long before immune systems developed in creatures, the pleasure principle existed. Based upon body parts that register and interpret feelings, these processes have evolved.

In the most complicated of all creatures, human beings, the brain and nervous system are the main pathways of conveying these survival processes. Thoughts, emotions, and good feelings instantly affect the body through mechanisms like neuropeptides and neuropeptide receivers.

The formula is basic: (1) sensations are experienced (2) when they are interpreted as good they are recognized as life promoting (3) the mechanisms that exist for such messages respond rapidly.

Not only did the pleasure principle precede the development of immune systems (because of its higher priority), it supersedes the immune systems actions. In other words the instantaneous response of emotions upon the body is much more rapid than immune system accomplishments. Furthermore, although one system is affected by the other, the pathways through which they accomplish their functions are not the same.

A few years ago a man in England made the news because he had been blind for twenty years and awakened one morning to find he could see. How?

In recent years a Miss America told of how she had one leg shorter than the other but through a faith healing the shorter leg grew to match the other one.

Were these changes brought about through the immune system and some kind of immune response? They appear to be accomplished through processes that were (1) swift (2) with built-in knowledge (3) accomplished through an intrinsic means to achieve their purposes.

The blind man's healing could have happened as the result of a highly charged dream ... perhaps a religious dream. These two seemingly unrelated healings could be achieved through the same processes. The "miracle" of seeing and the short leg growth are related through the life force, the emotions or the pleasure principle. They are accomplished through the basic forces that were so essential in the development of life in its earliest stages.

Religious experiences may be described with such mystical terms as divine, holy and ethereal. All of them are experienced as awesome emotions. They involve powerful feelings capable of changing body chemistry in dynamic ways.

The term that is less mystical is wholeness. Although it is also experienced with amazing sensations, wholeness is the term that can better help us get to a logical scientific understanding of a faith healing.

If religious experiences can be dynamic, life changing, life enhancing, health giving events, how could one better describe wholeness? What emotional words could one choose to better explain wholeness? One could use happiness, enthusiasm, pleasure, a sense of well being, etc.

But wholeness includes the mind, body and spirit. If we take the position that the spirit is our life force and the life force is energy that is the result of emotional interpretations, then wholeness is feeling great in a total way. All aspects of the body and mind are feeling totally well or whole.

In the last chapter I asked the question, "If the mind can make the body physically sick, can the mind make the body physically well?" Actually that question appears to be backwards. If emotional interpretations create the life force, and there are countless interpretations going on constantly, by far the vast majority of these physical sensations are positive and they are what run our bodies. Initially they are what keep us well. They are relative forms of the essential forces that created us in the first place. They are involved in the very processes of life. They influence the building of DNA of cells.

Every cell has its own DNA. Theoretically a total human being can be created from any cell in our body through cloning techniques. Every DNA has the potential knowledge for the rest of the body. The DNA does not change from birth to death but it involves expressing or suppressing different parts in the formation of the vast variety of cells in each body. It is DNA's active twin RNA that is responsible for carrying gene data from the nucleus to the cytoplasm of cells. In the cytoplasm it puts together proteins and *makes needed changes*. All of this is influenced by neurotransmitters and nueropeptides. And what directs them? The life force or the emotional interpretation of all thoughts, sensation, feelings and actions.

When I was searching through ancient religions of the Far East for descriptions of feelings that were similar to those I learned in healing episodes, I found some unusual terms. One described the spinal cord as a silver cord. Another suggested thinking of it as a white light.

One exercise that caught my attention was that of imagining the sensations of rolling a ball up the spine and out the top of one's head. Their literature cautioned about over-emotionalism when trying this exercise.

I couldn't comprehend how one could roll a ball out the top of their head since those feelings seemed beyond mind control. However, the sensations were quite similar to those of my worshipful feelings, so I learned to develop them. Also, they were related to the euphoria I experienced with the chiropractor's manipulation.

Both sensations rolled up the spine. Both approached the base of the brain, the hypothalamic region, in the same way. Both were capable of causing emotional sensations as the result of neuropeptides and their effect upon the hypothalamus.

When I learned the ball, spine exercise, the sensations resembled those of a specific prayerful attitude I used on a regular basis. There were feelings reaching upward and outward to God (the ball out the top of the head) which connected to the abdomen. These feelings always formed a line or cord.

The key was to recognize the similarity of sensations since they stimulated healing body chemistry. That is probably why over-emotionalism was not a problem for me. By then I was familiar with such feelings and they were wondrous rather than something to be cautioned about.

As for the ball rolling out the top of the head, it was not impossible. For one thing people who are in deep prayer often mentally reach upward to "God in Heaven". I found that there are sensations that can be involved in the devout exercise of reaching upward to God. They can be recognized and further developed. Furthermore, the ball out the top of the head didn't mean one would feel the ball after it left the body, what it did mean was the sensations of leaving the body were possible. One only has to think of how hot sunshine feels on the top of the head to recognize that there are sensations on the top of the bead. Or how about when one scratches their scalp or shampoos their hair?

I learned to do the ball up the spine exercise and often substituted it when I was emotionally exhausted or not feeling very religious. It has been valuable to me because it helped trigger religious feelings when I wasn't in the mood. It has worked for me over and over again.

As I became skilled at this technique I learned more about the healing chemistry involved in a faith healing. For centuries the solar plexus was thought to be the center of emotions. A few decades ago scientists recognized the hypothalamus as the seat of emotions and that ancient concept of an emotional center in the middle of the abdomen was temporarily changed.

What the ancients recognized, however, were the feelings. While the seat of emotions may be located in the head, there is no place where the body feels emotions more dramatically than in the solar plexus or center of the body. Deep feelings of laughter are the most obvious as one recognizes how the muscles and sensations move up and down. Fear and anger affect this area as all ulcer people know. Then there are sensations of wonder, awe, and joy.

Why does the mind's emotional interpretation affect the body in this area so much? Here are rich supplies of blood and nerves that act upon the vital organs like the liver, pancreas and stomach. These are essential for life survival.

Furthermore, rolling a ball up the spine causes the stimulation of all the endocrine glands which lie conveniently along this path: the ovaries or testis, the adrenal glands, the thymus, thyroid, pituitary and pineal gland. It is more than stimulation of these life-giving, fundamental processes of life. This also involves nerves and neuropeptides that make the healing difference.

This makes it easier to explain the revitalizing I experience in a religious exercise. It helps us grasp the energizing that Laura displayed after her prayerful episodes.

These understandings bring up another question. If emotional interpretations, the life force, are responsible for our front line of life and health and wellness, could it be possible to consciously overcome disease at that level? If a person, who has learned to enhance and employ faith healing exercises, uses these techniques from the onset of a disease, would the body fight the illness at that level rather than at the level of immune response?

Actually, looking at it from the other end of the spectrum, I think the question has already been answered. When numerous tests of healthy laboratory animals showed that they developed disease as the result of stress, when healthy humans have become sick and have had heart attacks as the result of too much stress and anxiety, the front line of health and wellness has been impaired. It is that positive emotional level of the life force that has been hampered. It isn't until this first level of life is impaired that the disease develops and becomes serious enough to require some kind of greater response from the immune system.

Yet it is at this first level that faith healings occur. It is in the area of relative forces that created us and are our life force that the mechanisms and chemistries for a faith healing take place. Can a person learn to consciously develop and use these energies? Obviously so, as most forms of meditation and wholistic medicine demonstrate. Certainly what I use and understand is a greater amplification of these processes.

At the University of Arkansas College of Medicine a thirty-nine year old woman amazed researchers by showing she could suppress her immune system at will. The test was done with injections of the virus that causes chicken pox and shingles. In the first test her body responded naturally with an increase in white blood cells and redness where the injection entered her skin. The second experiment was done while she was meditating. This caused a sharp reduction in white blood cells and there was much less skin reaction to the virus. Researchers in Arkansas were so impressed that they were curious to see if she could enhance her immune system through concentration.

Although mind-body research is being conducted in many of the major medical centers in the country, understandings are still coming in. While mind-body practices are as old as ancient religions, the understandings are conflicting.

To me the woman in Arkansas improved her infection through pathways that superseded her immune system. If she had suppressed her immune system, she would have invited more serious consequences from the viral injection.

If mind-body exercises can change the immune system response, is this why most doctors seem to believe that faith healings have been due to a psychosomatic illness or a misdiagnosis? If one of the traditional means used for medically diagnosing illnesses has been altered, what else are doctors to think?

"Spontaneous Healing" is one of the latest books written by Dr. Andrew Weil published on the subject of alternative approaches to medicine. He says the self-healing mechanisms in the body are much more than the immune system. He describes the healing system as a governing body with numerous divisions.

The immune system would be like the defense department that destroys invaders such as viruses and bacteria. According to Dr. Weil other parts of the governing body detect potential problems and handle them before disease develops. In other words at the front line of wellness, (my comment). Dr. Weil's training as a conventional doctor at Harvard is the background for his present occupation of teaching alternative approaches to medicine at the University of Arizona in Tucson. There he teaches students and fellow physicians how to combine traditional medicine with alternative treatments.

Holistic medicine always emphasizes that no matter what doctors do, it is the healing processes of the body that ultimately accomplish wellness.

When a person becomes involved with techniques outside of traditional medicine, surprising things can happen. While I have a healthy immune system and tend to let it handle routine things, I have had other serious illnesses which required all the help I could give. When I used mind-body concentration my immune system responses...tests that would normally be helpful in diagnosing and identifying a disease...have been known to be inadequate.

This raises questions that need to be addressed in this growing science. If an illness is fought at the front level of wellness and the immune system does not become highly activated, bow does one build up an immune response to a disease?

Lest this should sound like the mind-body, faith healing exercises are not desirable, one has to weigh the awesome achievements against the diagnostic inadequacies. With better understandings these difficulties can be worked out.

CHAPTER V

ANOTHER PUZZLE PIECE

When I was looking for the what, where and how of the sensations I experienced when I felt energized or was in touch with the healing energy, I studied a book on Human Anatomy published by Barnes and Noble. With clear pictures and descriptions it revealed all of the endocrine glands and body parts. In the early sixties I made note of the pineal gland, partly because it was in the pathway of the energy that I recognized and partly because it was listed as a gland whose function had not been established.

I did not know the role of this tiny gland in the healing mechanisms of the body but I felt sure it should not be overlooked. Not only did my concentration affect all of the known endocrine glands as it moved up the center of the body, but it was bound to have an impact upon this mysterious gland.

Human interest in the pineal gland has an ancient history. It has been considered to be the vestige of a third eye and has been thought to be involved in psychic powers. The pineal has been called a third eye because some of its structural components are similar to those of an eye.

For decades melatonin has been recognized as the hormone produced by this strange gland. Melatonin is now known to be valuable in the sleep/wake cycles of humans and other creatures.

The role of melatonin in wild animals has been more easily recognized because of other obvious cyclic functions such as hibernating, migrating and mating seasons that are essential for their survival.

In recent decades much research has been done on the pineal gland in humans. Results have been made known in medical journals and more recently in paperback books and on prominent television programs.

Melatonin is available over the counter in drug and health food stores and it is proclaimed as everything from a natural sleep aid to a source of enhancing one's sex life to a means of controlling the aging process.

What interests me, today, is the agreement by some researchers that the pineal gland is considered to be a "master regulator". Prior to this recent title of the pineal, the pituitary gland was known as the master gland of the body. A gland that is a master regulator suggests that its duties are not the same as a master gland and, indeed, some researchers are adamant that the pineal now supersedes the pituitary gland in its functions.

The hotly debated news about the pineal continues to be in the forefront of the news. In "The Melatonin Miracle" by Pierpaoli, Regelson and Colman, (reprinted with the permission of Simon & Schuster) the pineal is described as the master gland that oversees the operation of our other glands. Even more significant, from my perspective, is that "its influence is felt by every cell in our bodies".

Furthermore, the authors are confident that melatonin's primary benefit is in its ability to prevent "the downward spiral that leads to illness". This sounds like what I would call the front line of wellness.

The authors of "The Melatonin Miracle" have discovered that the job of the pineal gland is to regulate and harmonize the functioning of a number of bodily systems including the endocrine glands and immune system.

To approach this regulation from a different angle, Dr. Weil in "Spontaneous Healing" feels sure that if we could arouse the same kind of emotional healing response in the body as we do when we're in love, we could activate the healing system and possibly regenerate latent healing capacities in our genes.

If you have been following my perspective, you may be one step ahead of me at this point. Why do I emphasize religious emotion as a healing energy? Why does the energy flowing up the center of my body, reaching upward and outward stimulate the pineal body? Why does this exercise have an effect on any cell anywhere in the body?

Over thirty years ago I felt sure the pineal gland was involved in the disease reversal process but I didn't know how. Now the role seems more clear.

Gene research implies that if it isn't in your genes, it is impossible for your body to achieve. A January 1996 Newsweek focused on a different point of view. It said, "recent experiments threaten to dethrone DNA as surely...and as stealthily and unexpectedly... as little mammals replaced dinosaurs." It appears that genes can be altered after birth through early life experiences. Although DNA still holds the throne for body processes "its days may be numbered."

Gene research and gene therapy are among the modern "miracles" of scientific research. There are amazing and awesome developments in the making. But all of the facts aren't in yet and mind-body research just might have some surprising developments in this area.

There are several aspects of the pineal which fit into the mind-body exercises I have used. I have long noted that the healing energies Laura and I received as the result of our religious exercises were cyclic. They would last about 4 hours before additional help was needed. Before I had ever heard of circadian rhythms I was aware of a rhythm or pattern in these processes.

Also, because neither Laura nor I were permanently healed, I learned to think of these energizing/healing episodes as bringing the body functions back into balance. Because both cyclic and balancing exercises fall into the regulatory category, they would appear to be closely tied to the pineal gland. Critics in the melatonin debate say we are moving too fast. There is still a great deal to learn about melatonin and, since it is proclaimed as a powerful hormone, over the counter sales could prove unwise. Furthermore, many tests were done with animals and animals are not the same as humans. Certainly animals are quite different from humans in their cyclic and circadian rhythms.

More importantly, humans have minds with which we can shift or delay normal melatonin production. For example people who work night shifts, and those who are exposed to a lot of artificial light, alter melatonin production.

But the most likely reason human minds can alter melatonin creation is because we can think ... reason, create, learn, fantasize, believe (as in religious faith), invent and problem solve. Because of human minds we can choose when we eat, sleep, have sex, travel, etc. All of these things are not true for animals. If we look at melatonin as the master regulator and how its influence is felt by every cell in the body, it cannot be separated from the mind-body relationship and the role emotions play in this whole process of life.

However, because the greatest amount of melatonin is produced during sleep, it would seem that nature intended for melatonin to be minutely affected by thoughts and emotions... at least the conscious ones. Interestingly, much research has been done in recent decades, which indicates dreams are very valuable for our mental, emotional and physical health.

We all dream and it is the nature of dreams to be emotional. Experts have long connected dreams to our subconscious minds. One way or the other melatonin production cannot escape being influenced by what we think and what we feel.

Certainly the pineal is close to the hypothalamus where thoughts are emotionally interpreted. Nature has good reasons for such a placement.

I also know that all these years the location of the pineal has been in the pathway of my focus when I have concentrated upon the healing feelings or have used mind-body exercises for health purposes.

CHAPTER VI

COMMON DENOMINATORS

Where there is no vision, the people perish.
Proverbs 29:18

For decades highly trained and respected doctors of science and medicine have been demonstrating and supporting the value of different facets of religion. This has been done because of the mounting evidence that there are healthful aspects to a number of religious practices.

Faith, itself, has a significant effect on the lives of people who are under stress or are ill. Often medical science has bridged the major religions of the world, pointing out the values that are common among them. This has been done in spite of the fact that the roots of some of these religious practices are more than 5000 years old. On one hand the lengthy and consistent success rates of religious health practices have laid groundwork for acceptance in the medical community. On the other hand understandings of thousands of years ago and those of science today have seemed irreconcilable.

Still medical science has been doing an admirable job of building bridges. Nondenominational, factual reports have been their main focus.

Medical biofeedback practices that became known in the sixties have their roots in the meditation practices of Far East religions. Through biofeedback people have learned how to counteract stress, relieve migraine headaches, control pain and much more.

In 1975 Dr. Herbert Benson became famous for his book, "The Relaxation Response". At the time Dr. Benson was Professor of Medicine at Harvard Medical School and Director of the Hypertension Section of Boston Beth Israel Hospital. In the seventies stress was highly recognized as a contributor to disease. Numerous studies had demonstrated its negative effects on human health. "The Relaxation Response" was a direct outcome of religious meditation practices. With a few simple explanations, it became an obvious and welcome means to counteract stress.

Regardless of the cultural source, Dr. Benson related experiences of great religious leaders throughout the centuries who found peace through different forms of meditation. Beginning with Christian notables such as St. Augustine (A.D. 354-430), this author reviewed records of many mediators and their techniques of concentration which include ways of being connected to God. Martin Luther, Rudoph Otto, Fray Francisco de Osuna and St. Teresa were cited, as well as Gersham G. Scholem and Rabbi Abulafia of Judaism.

In the sixties concentration techniques called Transcendental Meditation became widely accepted and practiced in this country. With its roots in India, the value of this kind of concentration has been scientifically studied and its health enhancement qualities have been well established.

Yoga, now widely practiced in the U.S., has permeated Eastern religion and its philosophies. It is a method of meditation used in Brahmanism, Hinduism, Buddhism and others. The origins of these techniques precede the life of Christ.

With meditation exercises similar to Christianity and Buddhism, Sufism can be traced to the second century. It is the roots of Muhamadan mysticism.

By connecting concepts of God, religious words and sounds, Depak Chopra does an outstanding job of building religious bridges.

In "Healing Words" Dr. Larry Dossey, former chief of Staff of Humana Medical City, Dallas, and currently associated with the National Institutes of Health, describes ancient Greek and Persian philosophies that allude to the mind-body aspect of health and healing. Dossey also relates a wide variety of world religions and their healing philosophies.

The list goes on! One thing that is consistent about these medical and scientific efforts is the correlating of world religions through seeking common roles of health and healing. It is done with respect and little prejudice. In many ways medical researchers have achieved an exemplary appreciation for the oneness of God and mankind beyond any achieved within the religions of the world.

Change and openness does not come easily within any religion. Within religions there is more subjectivity than there is objectivity. Fear of change is not unusual. Over the centuries there have been reasons for this.

At one time Christian teachings seemed to have been impaled by Darwin's thoughts on evolution. Today there is little doubt that life on this planet has evolved. Sometimes the people who love a cat or dog, as though they were a family member, are the very ones who object the most to being related to more primitive forms of human life.

There are other scientific explanations that have had a significant negative impact on Christian teachings. The concept that creation was caused by a big bang and the millions of years of dinosaurs which seem to have no place in the Biblical creation story are but a few.

Now out of left field we see medical understandings about humanity, health and healing which are gleaned from religions around the world. Medical science has cut through religious rigidities and prejudices. They have assembled a core of worthwhile and amazing truths.

MY CHURCH

My church is more than another club
To which I can belong,
And pay my dues and volunteer
And sing some happy song.
It's more than another social group
Where I am entertained
Or join a cause or meet my friends,
(Though these things are attained).
My church is much, much more than these.
It's where my faith can grow
In a supportive atmosphere
With truths I've come to know.
It's where my heart's in tune with God...
A seeking, searching place,
A shrine wherein I worship God,
His wonders to embrace.
My church is unique above all else,
And may I not forget
That it's a holy, sacred house
Where deepest needs are met.

Jean A. Pentico

CHAPTER VII

MORE THAN FROSTING ON LIFE'S CAKE

The connections between medicine and religion are obvious. There are few things more important to a person than his or her health. Problems of health and the sufferings caused by disease are, in fact, one of the reasons religious faiths have been so valuable.

It is from ancient religious meditation practices that the modern techniques used in alternative medicine have evolved. Mental imagery, visualization and biofeedback are quite well known. In each of these practices there is a greater focus on thoughts than on emotions, even though it is most likely that the emotional interpretation of such thoughts is the reason body chemistry can be changed for health-and well being.

People are justifiably afraid of certain kinds of emotionalism. The healing emotion of religion needs to be clarified so that it isn't confused with hysteria, irrationality, etc. Unfavorable emotions can raise blood pressure, cause strokes, exacerbate ulcers or spastic colons and cause health damages.

Some of the latest research on emotion is revealed in "Emotional Intelligence" by Daniel Coleman. It explains in great detail the central role of emotions in life and survival.

According to Goleman the emotional part of the brain developed long before the logical thinking part. Emotions evolved in our more primitive roots where feelings of fear, anger and sex were essential for survival.

As our brains evolved and we could think, reason and use logic, connections developed between the emotional and thinking sections of the brain. With the thinking brain, emotions were still vital but they could be controlled through reasoning.

Because emotionalism preceded rationalization, there are some root areas where feelings still precede our thought processes. Researchers found a surprising and unexpected thing. In certain instances, those where we are likely to be emotional first and think later, there is a short cut within the brain... something like a back alley. In our early more primitive days this was critical. Timing was essential for survival.

Life saving, highly charged, emotional experiences are stored in that primitive part of the brain. Within a split second the brain can recognize these and cause the body to react. These age-old responses can backfire in our modern world. Acting before we use reason or rationalization can be destructive and anti-social. Uncontrolled anger is often involved in beatings.

Goleman says instantaneous responses are not always destructive. They can occur with laughter, joy and love.

There are several aspects of these more primitive reactions that are tied with healing experiences. Not only is that early part of the brain concerned with emotions but it is instinctively involved with human survival. Emotions, survival and body mechanisms are all part of of faith healing experiences as I understand them.

Medical science has carefully followed patterns of thoughts and emotions. It is now evident that the chemistry of emotions connects with those of the immune system. While this direct influence has long been suspected, identification of the process has been missing.

Psychoneuroimmunology is one of the latest and leading areas of medical science. This field links the mind, nervous system, hormone systems and the body's immune network.

Numerous researchers in this field are finding chemical messengers in both the brain and immune systems that are most commonly found in areas of nerves that regulate emotion. Goleman explains that Robert Ader, a psychologist, laid the groundwork for these understandings in 1974 at the University of Rochester. There, in the School of medicine and Dentistry, he made the revolutionary discovery that the immune system was capable of learning in ways similar to those of the brain.

A colleague of Ader's discovered strong evidence for a direct physical pathway whereby emotions influence the immune system. It is the autonomic nerve endings that directly touch immune cells where exchanges can take place.

By going a step further Felton demonstrated a huge drop in immune response of animals in which he removed some nerves in areas where immune cells are stored and made. He then subjected the animals to viruses and found their immune response was drastically lacking.

All those decades of experiments, which were conducted to prove that stress is involved as a cause in the development of disease, can be substantiated by pointing out many of the positive chemistries which are inhibited and/or the negative chemistries which are over-produced under stress.

Even more important is the recognition of the vital role positive emotions play in our health and healing. Because we now know that emotions preceded rational thought in our evolutionary processes, those kinds of feelings are at the core of our existence. In other words, "Emotions are more than the frosting on the cake of life. They are the nuts and bolts of our existence."

Religion, we assume, comes from higher more developed sections of the brain where through logic and appreciation we recognize our dependence upon a far greater intelligence in creation. But there are primitive aspects of these evolving religious thoughts and they have not been easily recognized nor appreciated.

It is the nature of primitive people to be highly uninhibited in their emotions. Nature has insured their chances for survival in this way. Uninhibited people not only show anger, fear, pleasure and love easily, but they are also more likely to experience awe in the presence of overwhelming beauty, wisdom and unfathomable aspects of life.

Awe is a common first step in religious experiences. Awe is a conscious recognition of human limits- -our finiteness. These feelings impact the emotional mechanisms and body chemistry. Because this emotion happens in relation to something or someone supremely greater than we, it involves a perspective which evokes immense admiration, appreciation and wonder for things like rainbows, sunsets and God.

Some definitions of this unique emotion include fear. Biblical religious experiences often involved fear. The fear aspect is relative to understandings in a person's society.

Feelings of awe can be followed by praise and adoration. This is not as easy as it seems, however. It is the nature of a "civilized" society to be inhibited in their emotions. Emotions are expected to be controlled. The emotions that can be freely expressed are largely dependent upon the society in which one lives. Thus it may be acceptable for two people to have sex the first time they kiss (as many movie and television shows depict) but the expression of religious emotion may be frowned upon.

If emotions are at the core of our existence (our life) and uninhibited emotions are not desirable, if medical science has repeatedly shown that suppressed emotions can be internally destructive to our health, what is the answer?

For much of this century we have measured people by their IQ. We have assumed an intelligent society is a civilized society. This has not been a very accurate way of measuring human qualities. Goleman points out that we literally have two brains; the emotional brain and the thinking one. Without the emotions that cause us to make essential judgements, life is lifeless. It is not the suppression of emotions that is the answer, it is the WISE use of emotions that is needed.

There are many qualities of life which help to insure success, health and happiness more than having a high intelligence quotient. The ability to relate to people, intuitive ways of recognizing other's feelings, knowing one's own feelings and communicating them well, are some valuable traits.

Not only is the wise use of emotion a vital part of human happiness, success and health, emotions dictate the production of body chemistry. Emotions have been crucial in the development and survival of life. This has been far more than the famous fight or flight phenomenon. From the evolving of primitive forms of life to the amazing human being, things that feel good and are life promoting have been emotionally interpreted in some form and noted in the genes. Likewise with negative feelings. Emotions have helped determine our physiological being. They have dictated that we see as we do instead of having the highly specific sight of birds or that our ears are on each side of our head, instead of on the top like many animals, and that we are capable of hearing the sounds that we can hear instead of the vastly greater scope of audible tones known to a dog.

Once we grasp the vital role of emotions in the evolving of human life, its development and survival, it is easier to recognize that a faith healing involves an emotional passion that is at the very basis of life and human existence. It is more than an emotional high; a religious experience has often been called a total mind-body episode. Humans may be the only creatures who know what a faith healing is. This is because we have the capacity to think in terms of the All of Creation, Allah or God. The thinking brain has the ability to encompass a greatness far beyond anything the primitive brain can grasp. In this awesome expanse comes a multiplicity of emotional feelings that highly impact the body chemistry.

This is the kind of passion Dr. Weil refers to when he says passion may be the thing that unleashes the latent genes of disease reversal in our bodies. Weil cites several instances where a new romance or passion reversed serious, even fatal diseases. Such healings are noted in medical research throughout the world.

Why is great, positive emotion healing? It is built into our body mechanisms for the sake of survival. If having a new lover can reverse disease, experiencing the wondrous, even overwhelming feelings associated with the Almighty are passions with a far greater potential.

This sounds like a *wise* use of emotions to me.

BEFORE GOD'S THRONE

Oh God of dinosaurs
And men Neanderthal,
Your wisdom overwhelms us.
Before your throne we fall.

Through eons of time and space
You practiced on it all.
And when it comes to man,
Before your throne we fall.

With beauty and perfection
Your people you enthrall.
In awe and admiration,
Before your throne we fall.

Yet more than all of these
When on your strength we call,
Your steadfast love surrounds us.
Before your throne we fall.

Jean A. Pentico

CHAPTER VIII

FAR FEWER FOOLS

It is fitting for the understandings of faith healings to be grounded in the basic principles and forces that created life in the first place. There is wisdom and perfection in these processes. There is awesome beauty and power.

All of these words we have used in relation to God. This is, after all, why Christians have always given God credit for faith healings.

Faith is a powerful phenomenon. The mind-body relationship is very complicated and amazing. When I was searching for relative forms of this energy, I found much had been written about highly skilled gurus in India who, through concentration, could make their bodies do bizarre and uncommon things. Walking on beds of hot coals with bare feet has been reported. Controlling the heart rate through concentration is another known feat. Lengthy fasts and many accomplishments considered to be odd by the Western world were described.

Since all humanity is part of God's creation, I explored healings by primitive medicine men and healings by witch doctors in covens. It didn't take long before I realized that both sides of the mind body relationship had to be recognized in order to understand the whole.

There were primitive people who, when they believed they had been given a curse, would become ill and actually die. Witches casting spells and witch doctors with magic potions could influence people's health for good or bad according to the power of the patient's convictions.

On the other extreme were devout Christians whose hands were known to bleed like those of Christ nailed to the cross. There were medical records of men whose stomachs grew to appear pregnant when their wives were expecting.

In recent decades, science has found chemicals produced by the body which have calming, healing, pain killing and mood elevating effects. Endorphins, dopamine, seratonin and melatonin are among them. Endorphins are known to be produced during religious experiences.

In the sixties the biofeedback machine was new on the medical scene. I was eager to experiment with one to prove what I had learned about mind-body techniques. When I had a chance to use a biofeedback machine the doctor said I was very good and asked if I would demonstrate for his class.

In an era when few folks understood these things, this was encouraging to me.

The common denominator of all of the above is energy created by thoughts, the mind (conscious and subconscious). They affect body chemistry and body cells.

There is always the risk when trying to describe something not generally understood by medical or religious people that words are inadequate. It would be easy for people who are experts in the field of biofeedback to concentrate on the feelings of rolling a ball up their spine and feel nothing but sensations of rolling a ball up the spine. The key here is to know what feelings to look for and to enhance them.

I would not have been able to succeed at these concentration exercises during the first thirty years of my life because I would not have known what feelings I needed to strive to achieve. It is possible that many people who have had deep religious experiences, such as those described as being born again or saved, would better understand the feelings. Yet there is no guarantee, since there are religious experiences others have known that I do not understand. For instance I have never talked in tongues, yet people in a number of branches of Christianity do it on a regular basis.

From the outside, a stranger must find Christianity very confusing. Although God, Christ, the Bible and the cross are common denominators, the diversity appears to be far greater.

On an even broader scale, someone who has not been able to believe in God must be convinced all religions are bewildering. Still it is amazing that wherever civilizations have sprung up on earth eons ago, religion was commonly found. Human beings who have the capacity to think and reason have always recognized supreme wisdom, beauty, power and perfection in creation. It is from this perfection we have come. We are part of this perfection and it is what sustains us.

It is appropriate, then, that these meager understandings of faith healings should lead us back to the principles of life which created us in the first place. The problem is not that there have been so many seemingly unrelated religions (for does anyone truly grasp God's greatness?) but there have been so many unanswered questions.

The more scientists learn about the principles of creation, the more we learn about the mysteries of God. The perspective may not always be what we have believed on the other side of the "glass darkly", but the beliefs have been well grounded.

It was more than the wonders of nature that made religion evolve during the early years of civilization. Along with faith in gods that were supremely powerful and perfect, came fear of evil forces that influenced and often controlled their lives. What resulted was a belief in good gods and bad gods.

Confounded by ignorance and fear (for sometimes the good gods had to be feared too) there was a lot of religious emotion. Emotion became a vital part of religion from its earliest days. Ranging from awe and adoration to fear and horror, religious emotion has been essential in its evolution.

As civilizations progressed in knowledge and wisdom, religion made advances. The progress was not fast and it was not easy. A person's faith is often the one stable force in an otherwise unpredictable society and world. Therefore it may well be the last thing people will change or want to alter. Because an individual's faith is a matter of their beliefs, it is largely under their control. This means a person's beliefs can often oppose logic and reason.

Changes in religions came only when an outstanding new insight brought fresh hope and could be accepted by many people. Then it needed to survive over a significant period of time.

In more primitive civilizations changes came at the risk of angering the gods. Even in our Judeo-Christian background we can see the fear of God as an important teaching. Undesirable human qualities were also attributed to our Biblical God because He was viewed from limited perspectives. Therefore, God was jealous, easily angered and vengeful...qualities that remained important in many of our Christian teachings throughout the centuries and into much of this century.

The more science has taught us, however, the more we have seen the perfection in creation. At the same time those things that we used to fear are no longer being viewed as punishment for human sin. Storms, earthquakes, fatal illnesses and human tragedies are not brought about by a judgmental God who is determined to punish sinning.

Modern science has brought us so far so fast that religiously our heads have been spinning. For instance, if there is the perfection of God in every atom in the universe, then it would appear that all things are perfect.

Certainly what we all view as good or bad is completely relative to our teachings or beliefs. While it would be an unlikely possibility for humans to believe all things that happen in the universe are perfect, especially when it comes to human behavior, we can better comprehend that all things repulsive to you or me may not be repugnant to others. A basic example would be spiders, snakes, roaches, slugs and worms. To some of us all of them might be disgusting, a few people could study them and find them fascinating, others might have a few of these creatures for pets and still others might be eating any of these critters as part of their regular diet.

My grandmother was so horrified of snakes that she couldn't stand to look at a picture of one. If she would come across one by surprise in a book, she was truly frightened. By contrast our niece has been known to handle and enjoy snakes.

In the Bible we are told that God looked over everything created and pronounced it good. Human beings have been struggling with that ever since.

It's true that we now understand the causes of things like tornadoes, floods, earthquakes, hurricanes and blizzards. They are the result of specific atmospheric conditions (or underground ones) and few people shudder in trembling at God's wrath as punishment through these calamaties.

We know diseases are caused by bacteria, viruses, parasites and specific things, but they are not the result of God's anger.

When it comes to human behavior, however, we still have a lot of problems. There is the concept that humans are sinful as the result of Adam and Eve's disobedience to God. Then there is the free will angle. We are told human beings were given free will, therefore, our destructive behavior, our disobedience to God, has been the result of our free will.

It was when we learned about the millions of years of dinosaurs, when we learned about the evolution of life from simple celled creatures that we became confused. It was the various forms of Neanderthal beings that preceeded us in our evolution that caused us to be in a religious turmoil.

We thought we had the understandings. We thought our religious perspectives presented creation, life and our sinfulness with proper points of view.

In reality the universe is vastly greater than anything Biblical authors could ever imagine. The evolution of life involved millions of years. In all of this was perfection and wisdom. Our knowledge, whether it be scientific or religious has always been relative to the times and what we could grasp or comprehend in a specific era.

Today we have come a long way in understanding creation and human life. The miracles and mysteries are dissolving all around us. Still the more we learn the more we realize there is to learn. The fact remains that we are the ones who are lacking in understandings. We are the ones with limited knowledge. And when it comes to human behavior, there is more than the concept of Adam and Eve and sin that determines our behavior and actions.

FINDING GOD

You can find God in a sunrise,
A rainbow or a setting sun.
You can find Him on a mountain
Or in children having fun.

You can find God in great music,
A hymn or a heavenly song.
But when you find Him in your heart
You know you can't be wrong.

You can find God in a snowflake,
A flower or a singing bird.
You can find Him in a raindrop
Or a baby's voice you've heard.

You can find God at a seashore,
Or a life lived well and long,
But when you find Him in your heart
You know you can't be wrong.

Jean A. Pentico

CHAPTER IX

IGNORANCE IS NEVER BLISS

The fact is all life struggles to survive. Until our last dying breath, life is making every effort to survive. This is programmed into our cells, our chemistry, our brains. Instinctively, subconsciously, primordially we are programmed to survive.

It has already been stated that many decades of scientific study have shown anxiety and stress to be involved as a cause in the majority of human illnesses. It should come as no surprise, then, that humans are instinctively counter-balancing this destruction.

People do this by following the pleasure principle. Pleasure, of course, is relative to each individual, the society in which they live, and the guidelines which they have been given or taught. Therefore, our good feelings are derived from a wide range of activities. What is pleasing to one may be repulsive to another. Likewise, what is sacred to one may mean nothing to another. Things that range from drugs to theft to opera or sky diving can bring pleasure to different personalities. We can conjure up good feelings of patriotism that include killing the enemy. We may feel good if we get revenge or "get even"... or we may thrive on helping others, being innovative or learning a trade, a profession or art.

What nature dictates is stronger than what humans attempt to order. This is especially recognized in our needs to eat, sleep, procreate and exercise. It is also noticeable on the small day to day levels of pleasure seeking. Snacks, cigarettes, pop, coffee, candy, chocolate, favorite foods, smells, music...the list is endless. Some of us become overweight because of our pleasure seeking, others become addicted to cigarettes, coffee, alcohol, and drugs. Pleasure seeking is best controlled when we learn early in life to find pleasure in discipline.

We are forced to make moderation a goal in all things but it doesn't always work. Most of nature regulates itself quite well. Humans are somewhat different. A lot of our behavior comes from who we are, what we have experienced in our lives and how we have used our minds and talents to solve our problems.

Nature is full of what we see as harsh, cruel realities but it is also full of perfection, wisdom and awesome beauty. Humans are the epitome of creation yet we are part of nature, just as nature is part of us.

Nature is made up of positives and negatives. From the tiny atoms that comprise all things in the universe to the solar system, the Milky Way and ends of creation, opposites are constantly at work. The same pattern of opposites is evident in everything from the electrons and protons inside all atoms, to the planets revolving around the sun, to the orbiting Milky Ways of the universe.

The earth is made up of positive and negative principles. There are acids and alkalines, darkness and light, night and day, hot and cold. These opposing forces are always balancing and counter-balancing, always controlling and regulating the mechanisms that run our universe, our world, our health and our lives. Since there are many exterior forces that influence our health and our lives, we are consciously and subconsciously involved in attempting to control our feelings and our actions in order to find some sort of balance.

If all creation is made up of opposites and opposing forces, why should we as humans expect that our life experiences be any different? Isn't it both the good and bad experiences that develop our character? Without ugliness do we truly appreciate what is good or beautiful? Without sorrow do we really know joy? Without winter, can we recognize spring?

In religion we sometimes believe we should be protected from the ugly and painful. In our religious faith we like to think God will shelter us and save or cushion our lives.

In reality there are positives and negatives everywhere. Without them we probably wouldn't exist.

Furthermore, God is not some super human being in the sky who plays chess games with our lives. Nor is He someone who makes the other team lose so that our team can win. These are limited human concepts.

Our problem has not been a lack of faith as much as it has been our religious confusion. Certainly religious beliefs are interpreted and influenced by the experiences of their writers and teachers. Because human understandings are restricted by our finiteness, there is imperfection in any religion.

Not long ago a minister made the statement that the walls of churches were no longer the greatest boundaries in religion. The problem is no longer what denomination we belong to. As human being, we have been breaking through those walls quite well. The division line now is more likely to be between the conservative and the liberal religious perspectives.

Modern science has propelled us toward liberal views while providing us with more proof of some of our ancient and conservative ones. We like to believe there is a reason and a purpose for all things, yet sometimes the reasons are very hard to see.

When scientists learned about the precision of atoms and how all things from here to the end of the universe are composed of this perfection, it should have reinforced our concepts of Supreme wisdom and perfection. Yet we were confused by the heartless behavior of humans and the pointless suffering we saw on earth.

Often we look to nature for perfection: a sunrise, a sunset, a rainbow, a flower. We tend to look at beauty as products of God but not ugliness. Yet ugliness is relative and it is obvious that God sees beauty in countless things that humans do not. Spiders, bats, slugs, maggots and worms are despised by many yet who can assume they are not beautiful in God's eyes?

Opposite forces have been pitted against each other in the development of history, scientific progress, understandings and behavior. Just as I do not like spiders or roaches, I am not going to like everything that I experience or encounter in my life.

Thinking humans are the only creatures who can reason, learn and create. We can appreciate and question. Some people argue that religion is a man-made thing, therefore, it is as easy to abolish as it is to make. That may be true of religion, but can the same be said of the beauty and perfection of creation? Whether we choose to be religious or not, the wisdom of creation remains.

Humans can live without religion. They may find love and purpose and happiness without the perspective of a higher power upon whom they depend. Yet every morning when they get up they have faith that the earth will keep on spinning, the sun will keep on shining, and that food and water will sustain them. They have faith that digestion, respiration, circulation and the functioning immune system will keep them alive and well. Without recognizing or admitting it they believe in a higher power.

Contrary to what many people believe, humans can be happy without religion. They can be loving, dependable, honest and trustworthy. What they do not have is the joy of religious experiences. They may benefit from religious holidays and profit from the materialism of them, but the special support of a community of believers would be missing.

The questions that keep some people from becoming religious are the same ones that plague us all. Why are there starving people? Why does God allow suffering children? Why are there tornadoes, hurricanes or floods that kill thousands ruthlessly?

Perhaps the ultimate faith is to love God so much that nothing can devastate us by comparison. Or maybe it could be better stated by saying

God loves us so much that nothing can devastate us. There are Biblical scriptures that allude to these things.

Someone once argued with me about the absence of some of my perspectives in the Bible. Her point was that if God wanted us to know these things, He would have made sure they were in the Bible. I think it could more accurately be said that we receive understandings according to the times in which we live and the era in which we are able to comprehend them.

As for why there is unfair and cruel suffering, we have already eliminated the ancient concept about sickness and tragedies being punishments of God. And since God is not some super human being in the sky who plays chess with our lives, it isn't a matter of letting anything happen, it is a matter of being.

GOD'S WEEDS

There are no weeds in God's garden.
Each has a purpose and place,
And I can't help but wonder
What that means for the human race?

There are no hated bugs nor worms
Who devour and deface.
Each has a part in creation;
Each has its own reason and space.

So in the greater scheme of things,
Where beauty and might embrace,
I cannot help but wonder,
What's the role of the human race?

Are we like weeds and critters,
Ordained by His Perfect Grace,
To fulfill creation's roles ...
Each in his own time and his place?

Jean A. Pentico

CHAPTER X

RHYTHMS

Primitive civilizations throughout the world embraced religion for thousands of years. In the beginning it may have been because thinking people realized how much they depended upon the wisdom in all nature. At the same time there was the element of fear because nature was also temperamental and destructive. By worshipping the mysterious forces that were in charge of all these things, there was a chance that people would gain the appropriate reward, such as being saved from floods, droughts or famine.

Remnants of those early religious principles are still evident in our beliefs today. But what began to happen, years ago, took an interesting turn. People started to realize that the act of believing became a vital force. Believing, it would seem, was perhaps the greatest facet of religion. With faith one could move mountains (at least personal ones), purify one's heart and even be made whole or well.

With the realization of the importance of faith, religious leaders began to incorporate into their teachings aspects that would enhance the faith of their followers.

In the early days there were food, animal and human sacrifices. Primitive rituals and ceremonies were performed. Oils, incense and music were added to their services. Stories of great faith became part of a tradition and they were handed down to each generation.

The object of these things has always been to enhance people's faith. It is faith that has been the basis for all religions and the source of religious acts. Faith is the energy of religion.

As civilizations evolved and beliefs progressed, some of the faith enhancing techniques changed too. The facets of religion that have been the most effective in increasing people's faith have survived the best.

Where faith is concerned, however, the doors are wide open. That is why in this part of the twentieth century, when we have made incredible technological advances in other areas of our life, we can still find people who believe in witches, burnt offerings, demons and punishments of God. Superstitions, which are easily incorporated into religion, remain in many faiths both in this country and around the world.

Because of the wide open doors, religious charlatans continue to thrive. One wonders how these people can survive in our sophisticated world.

Certainly, in spite of all our progress, people are still committing horrendous and horrible acts. In an earlier chapter I suggested that all creation is made up of opposite forces. Why should humans expect to be any different? This is a rather stark, cold and uncomforting observation. There is a more beautiful way to view these opposites of creation. Described as nature's rhythms, they are part of life. Rhythms are compared to breathing out and breathing in. They are like night and day, summer and winter, hot and cold. Rhythms are life giving, life enhancing. Rhythms have a purpose, a critical reason for being. There is a progression in nature's rhythms. They make up the dance of life, the evolving of creation. We are a part of it all. How can we not be?

Taken a step further, rhythms make up circles and cycles. These may be beyond our vision and comprehension...like our solar system that was not understood until we had the proper equipment to comprehend. In the same way human trials and tribulations, human pain and suffering may be beyond our vision and comprehension. Still, they are a part of the whole. They are a part of the dance of life...the dance of creation.

We influence our own rhythms. By counter-balancing pain and suffering with positive thoughts and actions we become part of the process...part of the dance.

CHAPTER XI

WHAT MIRACLES

"Miracles do not happen in contradiction to nature but only in contradiction to that which is known to us in nature,

St. Augustine

The more we learn about the supreme wisdom in creation, the more it becomes apparent that there are no miracles in "God's eyes". The dictionary describes a miracle as an event that surpasses all known human or natural powers and is ascribed to a divine or supernatural cause. Therefore miracles exist only to humans. We are the ones who don't have the answers wherever a miracle is proclaimed. Traditionally we would say our Creator knows even though we don't. Another way of expressing it would be to say there is more intelligence in creation than we have ever begun to comprehend.

Countless miracles have been understood over the years as they have been translated into scientific information and facts. A sunrise, a sunset, a rainbow, a flower, a mountain, a baby...all of these are awesome. Because most of their processes and components have been learned, we no longer look at them as miracles but as things that follow laws of nature and science. At the same time comprehending the processes of such things always multiplies the recognition of Supreme Wisdom in creation.

Understanding about oxygen, air and red blood cells explains why it is miraculous for a suffocating person to revive when he is given oxygen. Learning about vitamins, minerals, food and digestive juices explains why a starving person regains vigor when he eats food.

Because they are no longer viewed as miracles, it is tempting to deny that God is in all this. Still supreme wisdom, order and perfection have always been evident as we have continued to learn about creation.

Religiously we have come to believe God is in the heavens, that He created all things, controls all things and is perfect love. The modern view that says the universe is billions of years old, is made up of countless galaxies (measurable only in light years) and that there were 150 million years of dinosaurs before Adam and Eve, seems to make God far too remote. Even the Biblical descriptions given by Christ are inadequate to portray such an Almighty God.

Still, it is in the understanding of miracles that we have more facts and proof of a Higher Power, Supreme Wisdom and Omniscient Intelligence.

SIGNS

In my tears I asked God for a sign
A sign to show all would be well.
He said, "One sign? My child,
Don't you know?
You're surrounded by signs
Wherever you go!
If you would take heed
And look everywhere,
You'd see countless signs
That show how I care:
The sun that shines,
Stars in the sky,
Flowers that bloom,
Friends passing by.
Endless and timeless
Are signs of my love...
Infinitely more
Than the heavens above!"

Jean A. Pentico

CHAPTER XII

GOD CONNECTIONS

Religious people both in and out of Christianity have often found they could make a connection with the Wisdom of the Ages, our Higher Power, Allah or God. The effects have been known to be dynamic. Hearts have been warmed and lives have been changed.

Such an experience places one's life in a new perspective. Some call it a proper perspective. We are created with mechanisms to experience such an event. It is free. It does not depend upon money, deeds or penance. The gift of this potentially life changing, health-giving experience is already ours.

My first experience with this dynamic force happened when I shared a hospital room with an older lady of another Christian denomination. Between bouts of being placed in ice baths to bring down my dangerously high fever of one hundred six degrees I sounded afraid and worried. I would yell for the nurses. It was not a very nice situation.

My roommate asked if I was a Christian. This surprised me since I had attended church all of my life. Then she asked if I believed in God. I don't recall my answer but what I do remember is a small pamphlet she handed me with Christ's picture on the front. The words that stood out, and the only words I remember, were, "God is as close to you as your hands and feet and nearer than breathing."

I had more than an intellectual realization. It was a total mind-body experience.

Yes, I was ready. Yes, I was in dire need. You could even say I was ripe for the occasion. However, that doesn't mean the experience wasn't real or the feelings weren't dynamic.

It was with this new-found faith that I was hospitalized less than a year later for a diagnosis. I had a pain and pressure under my right ribs that limited my activities and movement. It was logical to start with a gallblad-der test. While I was hospitalized my problems exploded. A raw searing pain began moving through my chest and into my head. Swollen glands started forming all over my body...some in places I didn't know glands existed. For ten days various medical specialists were consulted to make a diagnosis. Confident that between my faith in God and my capable doctors I would have an answer, I regularly practiced my "healing feeling" rituals.

At the end of ten days my doctor came to me and said I definitely had something. They didn't know what it was, but it probably was a virus. With that, he announced that they were going to dismiss me from the hospital. I was dumbfounded!

I went home from the hospital. The swollen glands and health problems continued. My nervous system and bowels were drastically affected. It was the beginning of life-long breast lumps. My shoulder joints were permanently damaged. I could be active for only short periods of time before I would be forced to lie down due to the chest pain.

This began months and years seeking additional medical opinions from specialists in various clinics. It meant the return of many of the symptoms when my resistance was down, such as after having the flu. Often this would last for weeks.

Throughout all this time I had plenty of experience practicing the "healing feelings".

Early in my religious experiences I concluded that God was far greater than anything written, sung, painted, sculpted, or portrayed. In fact my convictions of this were so great that I was somewhat angry to think that such an incredible perception of God had not been revealed to me by another human being.

Furthermore, I felt showered with understandings. Feeling humble and overjoyed at the same time, I began collecting material and making notes to explain these perspectives. My top priorities were my husband, children and ailing health...not always in that order.

Paralleling these things were my religious perspectives. First of all God was real. Therefore, I concluded, God was in reality. I began looking at what was logical and real to explain my understandings. To me the God of creation, the God of Christianity, was everywhere, in, of and with all things. I was open to finding answers and explanations anytime, anywhere.

In the beginning I didn't realize this God of everywhere was a reference to an omnipresent God. If I had, I might have been discouraged by some insurmountable theological teachings.

I did have a sense, though, that believing God was real meant there were far less mysteries than we have accepted in the past. It meant there were no miracles in God's eyes- -only in ours.

Countless miracles of life, health, death and the universe have become medically and scientifically known in these four decades since this all began for me. There is little doubt that we are living in a unique era for mankind, not only scientifically but religiously.

HIS GREATER REALITY

I rarely say, "With God's help"...
It doesn't seem to fit.
With God who's omnipresent,
Such words bind and limit.

I think we have it backwards.
It's God who's in control.
We are simply helping Him
To reach some awesome goal.

When we make God connections,
We are the ones who see.
And we have merely tuned in
To His Greater Reality.

Jean A. Pentico

CHAPTER XIII

AWESOME EVOLUTION

Just as we can learn something about an artist by studying his works, we can learn more about God by studying creation. After all, most religious roots began with the recognition of creation's greatness. People have always worshipped gods because of the beauty, power, perfection and wisdom in nature. Our Christian worship of God relates to this. The book of Psalms is full of such songs of praise.

What we have learned in this century about atoms, solar systems and galaxies adds awesome dimensions to our cause for worship. What we have learned about evolution enhances our perceptions of creation as well as the greatness of God. Instead of being a destructive concept in opposition to the Biblical creation story, evolution is the link between a universe of galaxies that we know exist and the creation story as the Biblical authors believed it existed.

Evolution is much more than opposing forces coming together and interacting. Evolution moves forward in cycles and circles of time and space, progressing, honing and perfecting all things. All people, all actions, all nature is interrelated. Nothing is truly separate. "No man is an island." When events or creatures appear to be haphazard or isolated, it is only because our finite perceptions keep us from seeing the larger picture. Isn't this what we have always said about God's perspectives versus man's?

Understandings that can broaden our religious thinking as the result of learning from principles of evolution have been illusive. Still, they are numerous. For instance, it is clear that opposing forces such as hot and cold, acids and alkalines, light and darkness are all valuable or "good" in God's eyes. Since goodness exists in both facets of all these kinds of things, there is endless goodness beyond anything previously recognized. It is easier to see the values of nature, its interrelatedness, and the wonders of each specie depicted by modern television on this subject. We can see a purpose and reason for creatures once despised and condemned.

With common patterns evident throughout creation, with specific designs repeated in concrete things, isn't it likely that human lives and progress are also following cycles in which perfecting and honing are taking place? Certainly this appears to be true in scientific progress such as in medicine, astronomy, geology, archaeology and others.

It should be noted that some things progressing in cycles are so huge that they seem to be standing still. For example the sun is rotating through orbit at 140 miles a second but it appears to be stationary. If this is true with something as important as the sun, are there other illusions that exist and facts that we need to know to be in touch with greater realities? Not only in science but in religion?

When opposing forces come together, a third quality often results. The new quality may flourish and be strong or deteriorate and die, depending upon the wisdom of these principles. Similarly, ideas, understandings and teachings survive or die depending upon their wisdom and strengths. In other words human progress follows evolution in these respects. There has been far more wisdom and perfection in these processes than we have imagined.

Built-in controls exist from the electrons and protons inside of every atom to the balancing of planets in the galaxies of the universe. All things come into being through the honing processes that interact and evolve. Supreme Wisdom exists in these patterns. What we have believed because of faith alone in the past is now acceptable because of what we can see and know...because of realities we have learned from the evolutionary processes.

CHAPTER XIV

JUMPSTARTING LIFE

Wisdom is the principle thing; therefore get wisdom: and with all thy getting get understanding.

Proverbs 4:7

I have been close to death a number of times and for me the feelings are not easily forgotten. I know the difference between feeling exhausted and feeling deathly tired. I know the difference between being very sick and deathly sick.

If I have something common such as a bad case of the flu, I never flippantly say, "I could have died." I have too much respect for life to be that casual.

Not long ago I was pulling weeds on a rocky bank in our yard. My foot slipped, twisted and popped. In agonizing pain I crawled to the nearest step and evaluated the situation. Alone and seemingly helpless, I rapidly shifted to healing energy. With this focus it wasn't long before I could hobble to the house. The next 36 hours involved more pain, more concentration, a call to the doctor, ice packs and more pain. A day and a half after the injury my foot was x-rayed. There was no evidence of a break. I then put my full weight on it and have had no trouble with it since.

Recently a look in the mirror showed my nipples inverted and, upon examination, a whole new series of palpable breast lumps. These kinds of things have changed through my mind-body exercises before, so they were shifted to top priority in concentration efforts.

Often a noticeable change in the structure of such lumps occurs while I focus healing energy upon them so I know this works for me. However, I firmly believe in mammograms and have them done on a regular basis. Sometimes this has been after an extraordinary episode with breast lumps. Then the confirmation that these problems were benign has always been prudent and welcome.

Obviously there are relative forms of useful mind-body energies. In the first chapter I referred to anger and adrenalin as the chemistry that brought me out of a near-death experience. It was after I had recognized the value of emotions as the core of life and healing that I consciously exercised them in other near-death and less life-threatening instances.

One mind-body exercise I employ is commonly learned in biofeedback training where extra energy is focused upon a specific location. This can raise the temperature of that area and increase its blood flow. Such an exercise involves no obvious emotion (although one should always keep in mind that all thoughts are emotionally interpreted).

There is a general faith healing exercise I practice in which worshipping God with praise and adoration brings tears to my eyes and internal sensations of joy. I utilize this most commonly because it has the widest range of possibilities and I have had the most success with it. It is the basic exercise from which all other relative forms of my mind-body controls have evolved.

The next exercise is along the same lines and combines the two previous techniques. Because it is highly concentrated, it is the most powerful form of mind-body energy that I know. Since I am self-taught it has sometimes taken months to employ. My carpal tunnel problems were like this. I was at the point of needing surgery to prevent the loss of use of my hands. Relief for them came when I finally learned to add healing emotions to the focus of energy in order to expand the space that cramped the nerves running to my hands.

In an earlier chapter I mentioned a healing exercise in which I focused on the sensations of rolling a ball up my spine. I saw this technique as a relative form of the general faith healing exercise. At first it sounded sacrilegious until I realized it was evidence of the God-given healing chemistry we each possess.

It is no coincidence that I often seem to see the doctor after the fact. That is after I have achieved improvement, I show up at a doctor's office. Obviously this can present problems. Coordinating medical help with what I have learned about the body's healing energy, and a person's ability to tap into this God-given force, has not been easy.

At this point in time, in the era in which we live, that is to be expected. But mind-body understandings are growing so rapidly this will not always be the case. More and more information is available through alternative forms of medicine.

I like channels such as biofeedback because the techniques are accepted by most doctors, they are available to anyone who cares to learn them and their instructors are most likely to be trustworthy and dependable. Besides, a person could be missing essential medical attention. Charlatans do exist and there is a risk when branching out to other channels.

Of course the faith healing energy I have described is available to anyone and is at the top of my list. The third category where I combine biofeedback concentration with the emotional chemistry of a religious experience is less well known but it is not difficult to comprehend because through biofeedback a person can learn to direct energies within their body. The next step is learning to direct the healing energy of a religious experience to your greatest point of need.

Because people respond with different degrees of emotion, and because body chemistries are not exactly the same for all people (although they exist in relative forms) I think it is important to emphasize once more that the category of faith healings is open ended. While I may need to repeat healing exercises many times on a ritualistic basis, someone else could have a complete and instantaneous healing. I mentioned in an earlier chapter that I do not claim to understand all kinds of faith healings, however, it is pretty certain that the disease reversal chemistries that work in one kind are the same ones that operate in all types of faith healings. There may be different sources and pathways, but when it comes to the body, nothing new enters it to do the healing.

I learned mind-body exercises forty years ago out of a dire need and an incredible faith. Through analyzing where and how I experienced religious healing-feelings I learned to duplicate the sensations. I have successfully repeated these exercises countless times over the years.

As great as they are, I still do not use them for the common cold, flu or most types of infection. These are areas in which I haven't learned the specifics needed, and judging from the lengthy time it took to learn how to deal with my carpal tunnels, it is wiser for me to get medical attention when needed.

There are three kinds of disease reversal exercises I have practiced when feeling gut-level, deathly sick. In such a situation there has not been a specific spot upon which I could focus so the worshipful religious sensations have been my first choice.

We have a collection of tapes and records of music that I find inspiring and spiritually moving. These are used in different forms and settings to gain fresh perspectives and elements of surprise. The car stereo, a tape player with ear phones, a home stereo and record player are commonly used. Radios bring nostalgic and inspirational music. Music from the Mormon Tabernacle Choir to Bill Gaither's vocal band could not be any better if the heavens had opened up and choirs of angels were singing.

There are wonderful inspirational moments at church or as the result of televised religious services and programs but when a person is trying to get well, it is useful to have inspiring materials at their fingertips. Music is best for me. *Other times things like scripture, poetry, or nature bring sensations of inner joy.*

There is something amazing about religious emotion that is healing, but sometimes a person can feel so sick that it is very difficult to have such a positive focus. In Dr. Weil's book are described forms of energy which I have found useful. They are related to religious feelings because of the gut-level sensations involved.

It seems obvious that all of these exercises are producing some of the same healing chemistry. Dr. Weil describes the breathing exercises as bringing oxygen to the nervous system. Therefore, it seems to me, it is very likely that one of the aspects of a faith healing is the enrichment of the autonomic nerves with oxygen. While Dr. Weil describes a number of breathing exercises that are health promoting, there is one that I commonly use. It involves breathing in and out rapidly causing sensations to be experienced at the diaphram (gut-level) and at the base of the throat. This is not relaxing nor calming. Since it energizes the central nervous system, I find it helps bring body chemistries back into balance. I have often found relaxation easily follows this balance.

A relaxation technique I have often used in the middle of the night is to copy my husband's breathing patterns in his sleep. His breathing emphasizes exhaling. *This appears related to an exercise Dr Weil describes where exhaling is seen as the beginning of each breath cycle.*

I learned long ago that most forms of alternative techniques used in Holistic or Wholistic medicine have been learned through the study of natural healing processes in other areas of life and health. That is why all of this ties in so beautifully with religious healings because it is from the Wisdom of the Ages that we are drawing upon in each instance.

While oxygen enrichment of the nervous system may be part of the faith healing experience, it is likely to be only part of the picture. In the sixties when I started on this journey, I became aware of enzymes manufactured within the body which are highly specific. At the time, emzymes were being added to laundry soap. They had become a household word. It is their high specificity to change one factor of a tissue without harming another that made enzymes an excellent candidate for having a vital role in healings.

Then there are new nerve and brain chemistries that are being discovered all the time. We know they exist, it is only a matter of time before the whole faith healing picture is unraveled.

My concern is the countless people on the other side of the mystery who doctors see every day. Their faith is sustaining them through serious, even fatal illnesses. They do not know why some days they feel better than others. They do not know the role emotions play in their health. In fact most people view how they feel somewhat backwards.

If they feel physically well they are likely to be on a higher level of positive emotions. Of course medications or other physical or mental therapy could be the cause of their physical improvement. These things are likely to result in a happier patient and this is reality. At the same time their faith and the kinds of heartfelt emotions described a number of times in this book can make a difference in changing their physical ailments.

Interestingly, it is when a person is in dire need that his or her true emotions often surface. This is exactly why it is so valuable for people to know what it is that can make a healing difference.

To imply this healing energy is available only for Christians or religious people is too simplistic. Heartfelt emotions can be healing for anyone. We are all created with such mechanisms. There are different degrees and different kinds.

I know what kinds work for me and they have been from the pure river "of the Water of Life".

CHAPTER XV

POWER PERSPECTIVES

Not long ago I visited with a doctor of alternative medicine. He asked what imagery or visualization techniques I used in mind body exercises. When I told him I didn't use any he seemed surprised.

The fear that some doctors of alternative medicine have, where religion and faith healings are concerned, is religion places too much control in God's hands. This suggests the person is not in charge of his or her health condition. Mental imagery and visualization specialists often emphasize the control patients can have over their own health problems.

There is a perspective that I find helpful in this controversy. We need to go to the heart of the issue--our concept of God. If we think of God as a super human being in the sky who controls all forms of life and creation from afar, we are indeed limited.

If our forefathers believed in God when they could only see beauty, perfection and goodness in parts of life and creation, it was because they had a deep faith. How much greater should be our faith when we can comprehend that perfection exists in every atom of the universe? How can we doubt that wisdom reigns supreme when we understand there is intelligence in every cell? How can we doubt that we are part of Universal intelligence or that Supreme Wisdom is in, of and with each of us?

Each breath we take,
Each day we wake,
Each mile we walk,
Each step we make,
We are at one with Supreme Wisdom.

That is a humbling realization. We cannot be separated from Universal Perfection. We cannot be separated from God.

The problem is we have been a small handful of people on the planet Earth who, for a relatively few thousand years, have been trying to understand the incredible universe which surrounds us. Relative to the many billions of years the universe has existed, the 250 million years dinosaurs lived on Earth, and the 65 million years that have lapsed since then, we are little more than a grain of sand in the sands of time.

For a mere few thousand years in this vast eons of time, humans have been in awe of creation, have pondered its infinite wisdom and have questioned our human role in it all. Our efforts have been very admirable.

Mankind's attempts at religion have been quite commendable. Even so, in the greater scope of creation, they are like a single rainbow in an eternity of time.

The truth is human beings have sensed, felt and believed they had a connection with this incredible Intelligence. In the depths of our being we have experienced a special kind of awe, joy and a "Divine Presence".

Because feelings of a Divine Presence are fleeting, because perfect goodness has not always been easily recognized, this Infinite Intelligence has seemed to be distant. God seemed to come and go, making it necessary to reach out to Him. On one hand we have acknowledged His presence within us and on the other hand we have believed He was other than, above or outside of life as we know it. The confusion has caused endless problems. In efforts to maintain forms of stability, the Bible has been the epitome of our religious teachings and Christ has been the epitome of our man, God relationships.

These teachings have been the core of our Christian faith. They have often made the difference between life and death. They have also made the difference between sickness and health. Our religious faith brings peace, comfort, joy and strength. In short, our faith moves personal mountains.

Still our teachings are minute in the greater realm of creation. Little wonder that other world religions have found God connections in other ways. St. Augustine believed it was an instinctive need deep within human beings to realize this man/God relationship.

Actually the bond has always been there. It is in every cell of our being. Through the conscious act of seeking and the sincere desire to know, the door is opened for us. This is more than an intellectual process. It is more than absorbing and acknowledging some teachings. This involves feelings and emotions.

We have used words like Almighty, Divine, God, Lord, etc. All these have been human efforts to verbalize a greatness far beyond anything we could comprehend. We have written and sung amazing songs. Centuries of scholars, scientists, professors, anthropologists, theologians and countless others have attempted to proclaim the Wisdom of Creation. But it is vastly greater than any of these. God is beyond our efforts at words. Yet words are what we are forced to use to continue communicating our perspectives.

Some things are greater than words. They existed before words. They are at the center of our being, the roots of life, the core of our existence. They are feelings and emotions. Feelings of a connection with God, a oneness with Supreme Wisdom, a Divine presence...these are greater than words.

With precision in every atom and intelligence in every cell, faith becomes an extremely positive force in healing. It does not place too much control in God's hands. The control has always been there. Religion does not take control out of our hands. It recognizes and synchronizes our thoughts and minds with the Supreme Wisdom that already exists. Faith unites our conscious energy with the intelligence in every cell created to be constantly at work for health and survival in each of us.

In mental imagery and visualization, feelings become important. By imaging a peaceful country scene, feelings of peacefulness can be experienced by the body. Other visualizations can picture body parts healing. Through these processes bodily sensations enhance the production of chemistries which build wellness.

While I do not use visualization in mind-body exercises, or picture anything, I use my mind to create sensations. Instead of going the route of mentally picturing something to achieve sensations (which are then a by-product of visualization), I focus on the feelings in the first place. The energy is stronger and the potential for enhancement is far greater. In a way you could say, "I go for the gold."

SCIENTIFIC INFLUENCES

Scientists have thrilled and amazed us
In diverse and marvelous ways.
From secrets of cells to transplants,
They've lengthened our lives and our days.
But one thing we ought to remember
As we reap these awesome rewards,
They didn't invent these marvels,
They borrowed from nature's vast hordes.
Sometimes the issues get muddled,
Like the beginning of life and its end.
And although we have ravaged life's secrets,
It's God on whom we depend.

Jean A. Pentico

CHAPTER XVI

COMING FULL CIRCLE

Recently I watched a program on Public Television in which Alan Alda interviewed various researchers on some of the latest understandings regarding the workings of the mind. One portion especially interested me because it showed messages entering the brain, being emotionally interpreted and then scattering to different areas of the brain where similar experiences have been recorded. There they were compared with past events of the same nature.

Interestingly, experiences that have greater emotional involvement are recorded with a higher level of priority. This is in keeping with the higher level of emotions needed for survival in fight or flight, procreation and hunting for food, etc.

When the human body and mind are studied it is easy to forget that all parts of our body mechanisms evolved because they successfully helped us to survive. This parallels information in earlier chapters such as THE PLEASURE PRINCIPLE and MORE THAN FROSTING ON LIFE'S CAKE.

Medical science now knows that when we are sick, such as with an infection, the body responds in more ways than the development of a fever and an increased production of white blood cells. The entire mind-body responds to a health crisis.

That is why, when we have the flu, we eat less, move less, sleep more and show less interest in our usual pleasurable activities. We perceive our environment in a different way.

Such behavioral changes are very elaborate. Research at Louisiana State University Medical Center, France's National Institute of Health and Medical Research and our National Institute of Mental Health describe these life processes.

Through animal studies scientists are learning more about such pathways. The vagus nerve appears to be involved because it carries information from the brain to the heart and other internal organs. The brain and the immune system communicate as well.

It is significant that highly positive emotions are often involved in religious experiences. Since highly emotional events are recorded in the brain relative to survival, and positive religious emotion enhances wellness and healing, this means these connections are automatic and highly prioritized.

We know faith is automatic and occurs on countless levels prior to a conscious development of religious beliefs. Therefore physical mechanisms for wellness relative to faith are already in our bodies. They are in our genes.

It is because of an unconscious faith that a mother rescues her child from a burning house. It is because of faith that a man fights for his country, a child is saved from drowning, a pilot safely lands his troubled plane or a doctor saves an infant's life.

We give them additional words. We say they are acts of bravery, courage or skill. Yet subtract faith from any of these scenarios and where would they be? It need not be a confessed faith in God (for countless people truly don't know what they mean when they say they believe in God) but it is a belief in something more than themselves...something much greater than who or what they perceive.

We have faith each morning that the sun will remain in orbit or that digestion, respiration and circulation will sustain us. The list is endless.

Faith is deeply rooted, often unquestioned and sometimes unexplainable. It is at the very basis of human actions and being. One need not be religious to have faith or perform acts of faith. Neither does one need to be religious for faith healings to take place.

Interestingly, rather than being the rare oddity we recognize faith healings to be, they are constantly taking place on some level for health and healing all of the time. This is that front line of wellness referred to in an earlier chapter.

Religious feelings involve special sensations. They appear to be superior to routine feelings. Divine and holy are words that are commonly used. This keeps them in the realm of mystery and mysticism.

Yet in attempts to duplicate these special feelings I learned mind-body exercises which resemble them rather well. This is once where I use mental imaging. Through imaging an internal sensation of fluorescence in the solar plexus and chest, awesome feelings resembling those of holy sensations occur. If they are combined with other mind-body exercises described in earlier chapters, the feelings are amazing.

We know there are creatures in which fluorescence is common, such as fireflies, glowworms and creatures of the deep sea. Phosphorus is an essential mineral for their glowing.

There are several kinds of phosphorus. Phosphorus is an essential mineral in our bodies. Its level of importance is parallel to that of calcium.

We may not glow like fireflies but we can experience certain glowing sensations. They impact our body mechanisms for healing. Minerals are an essential part of these processes.

The earliest formation of life for each of us preceded pregnancy and the nine months in our mother's womb. The information in our genes began eons ago in the early evolving processes of life. Throughout the ages, those things conducive to our survival stayed recorded in our genes.

An unconscious faith has been part of life from its earliest beginnings. It is present in all living things. One could say life believes in life. Only in humans do we identify faith. Only in humans do we enhance, embellish and develop it.

It is possible that the feelings involved in faith healings tap the very core of the recorded sensations that created life in the first place. In a literal sense we may be in touch with the processes of life. It would be appropriate to say we are in touch with our Creator. A healing could literally be a form of being made whole.

Faith healings, then, are not something outside of, other than or beyond reality. Faith healings are of the real world.

THERE IS A POWER

There is a power surrounding us
To which we can relate.
It gives us strength and courage
No matter what our fate.

There's beauty and perfection
For us to know and see,
And it can bring us endless joy...
For it is vast and free.

There is a wisdom in it all,
Beyond our human skills.
It comes from God who gave to us
Life, love and human wills.

Jean A. Pentico

CHAPTER XVII

A REALITY CHECK

Today, as I walked to my car near a local shopping mall the sun shone brightly, mounds of snow were melting and winter birds were happily singing. Sand, remnants of the winter's protection against ice, crunched under my feet. My senses enjoyed the perfection of the moment.

Life should always be like that- -moments of perfection. I have been tempted to think that it is.

Someone else might have found the sun too bright for their eyes, the birds too noisy and the sand under their feet a nuisance. It is all relative to who we are, what we have experienced, what we believe and how we respond.

This is true whether it is an ordinary interpretation of a sunshiny moment, our religious beliefs, our political perspectives or any other aspect of our lives.

This does not mean sorrow, suffering, pain and heartache don't exist. Neither does it mean nothing should be changed where human actions are concerned. We can, however comprehend that there are reasons for all human actions. Even those that are horribly senseless occur because of someone's deep hurt, ignorance or the deprivation that helped form their actions and personality.

When we get beyond prejudice and blame, when we move beyond accusations and revenge, we know explanations exist. We have trouble seeing the bigger picture. That's part of our humanness. If we could see the broader view, "God's View", I suspect we would see life and all creation moving along perfectly in tune.

Throughout these chapters I have alluded to such a perspective a number of times. Still, it is a concept I have not been ready to accept.

It is one thing to say all creation is composed of perfect atoms. It is an enormous leap to say all creation is perfect. Even so, in the broader view, in the very basic principles of the universe, we know that all things continue to hone, perfect and create. The processes can be hectic, powerful, destructive, amazing, beautiful, awesome and incredible.

That's why faith is needed. That's why we need to emphasize the beautiful, awesome, amazing and good so that we are not overwhelmed by or discouraged by those things that are ugly, painful and seemingly destructive.

Destruction is also relative. By overcoming pain and horror through faith, people can become stronger, wiser and enlightened. We are all a part of creation. We are all a part of the bigger picture. Little wonder that we can be confused. Little wonder that we don't always understand.

Having grown up within Christianity I am well aware of the diversity of interpretations that exist. There is a honing and evolving going on in these opposing beliefs. It has been slow and difficult. Many of the disagreements have covered numerous centuries. Yet where strong truths arise and significant numbers of followers can agree, the truth survives.

For more than fifty years I have lived in many places and been exposed to a variety of Christian interpretations and teachings. There are advantages to all this.

I recognize that there has been growth, change, progress and evolving of understandings. For instance, when I was young and studied world religions we pointed out the differences. Today the trend has been to cite the similarities. When I was young we emphasized the differences in beliefs of various Christian churches. Today we often work together with common purposes and goals.

Once we recognize and accept this is how "God works" we can speed up the procedure. Like faith healings and the synchronizing of one's mind with the body's healing mechanisms, the course can be greatly enhanced.

Still I know there are hordes of people who go through the motions of being religious and have little conviction of what they are doing. I also know there are vast numbers of folks who have difficulty accepting our traditional Christian beliefs. For these reasons I submit:

MY REALITY CHECK LIST

1. Religion...the worship of a God or gods with the purpose of building faith.
2. Faith...the ability to believe in powers greater, wiser or stronger than oneself. Faith brings hope, courage, strength, peace and sometimes joy.
3. God...Supreme Wisdom, our Higher Power, Universal Intelligence.
4. Sin...destructive actions aimed at fellow beings. Today this might include fellow creatures and nature.
5. Righteousness...extreme goodness in people relative to religious beliefs.
6. In God's hands...in the wisdom, perfection and order of creation.
7. In God's eyes...in the broader view, the Greater Reality.

8. Heaven...the highest place of existence, elevated in our thoughts and beliefs through religious teaching.
9. Heaven on Earth...when goodness prevails on earth or when understandings reign on earth giving a reason and purpose for all things.
10. Hell...not knowing or understanding about God, being outside of or below the joy of religious faith.
11. Angels...mythical winged people symbolic of purity and goodness.
12. Spirits...an ancient term given to energies and forces not understood.
13. Christ...in Christianity the epitome of man/God relationships. Christ brought a central focus to the diverse concepts of God. His emphasis on the incredible caring nature, "love of God", has been revolutionary. It has changed lives throughout the world.
14. Holy Spirit...the recognition of God's energy in lives, churches and religions.
15. Faith Healings...bringing body mechanisms back into balance by impacting the built-in healing mechanisms through faith.

This list is different from what I might have written thirty years ago. That is because the world has become smaller, access to understandings about science, other lifestyles, nature, other religions and peoples is easily accessible.

Animals defecate. Leaves decay. These things form rich soil for plants to grow. Some plants feed our bodies. Some manufacture oxygen for us to breath. All things are interrelated and interconnected.

All people are at one with nature and the Whole. Each of us is part of the Greater Reality, God. All are worthy of respect and appreciation.

GOD'S WISDOM

Other men have been named Jesus;
Other men have claimed virgin birth.
Other men have been crucified.
Countless men have walked this earth.

Other folks have been great teachers.
All humans are children of God.
Other folks have healed sick people.
All these paths others have trod.

It is the God of the Ages
Who made it Christ's destiny
To best reveal God's nature
And His love for you and for me.

Jean A. Pentico

CHAPTER XVIII

IF I HADN'T BELIEVED

It is always more useful to have mysterious processes demystified and replaced with understandings in the real world. When something is a fact, it's easier to believe and can become far more common and beneficial. When a concept is mysterious, the truth can be misinterpreted and embellished. It can be glorified and even deified. No one can argue against it because it has an aura of otherworldliness. There is no proof, even though there is belief and faith. Therefore the mystery is propagated and sometimes distortions go with it.

That may sound a bit anti-religious but I would like to suggest there is a third perspective. We are in an era where we have been understanding and accepting facts that our forefathers believed on faith alone. We are in an era where the heavens have been opened up for us and understandings abound.

Christian faiths vary in their emphasis on this Biblical prophecy. Some take it literally. Others place little emphasis upon it. There is a popular hymn that says, "He has promised He would open up the Heavens". Because it hasn't happened within an hour, or even a day, we have been missing it. Yet in the broader view, in "God's eyes", the time factor is more like a single day. The understandings about life, health, survival, social interaction, international peace, environmental respect and religious perspectives have been here for years. The answers have been evolving, honing and perfecting for some time now.

When we haven't been able to understand or couldn't comprehend, it has been necessary to rely on symbolism and traditional teachings. When we haven't had the answers, when we needed incredible faith, we have built upon and enhanced what we have hoped for, desired and believed in the past.

Over thirty years ago I had gained an amazing faith and an incredible need. Fortunately my faith preceded the need. Most of my religious faith has come from Biblical teachings and the examples of faith my parents and elders have demonstrated.

Still, there were too many blank spaces. What I experienced and what I required were not available through my religious heritage. In the beginning I did not know whether I could live three years. I knew my religious exercises were profoundly affecting my wellness but more answers were needed.

Some of them I found in nature. In nature I could relate to concepts of God that were missing in my religious training. When I trusted nature, I was trusting God.

Initially the healing feelings brought regenerated health for short periods of time. When I recognized the cycles, they resembled those of an infant. By eating every few hours, taking short naps in cycles, and doing the healing feelings when needed, I was able to function. This left valuable periods of time to do what was necessary.

From the beginning I was aware of a basic rule: either the mechanisms of life were in control or there were interferences in those forces. Clearly, my mind exercises enhanced the life mechanisms. This I had demonstrated often enough to be convinced.

Early in the process I realized definitive answers wouldn't be found in medical schools, theological seminaries nor in my heritage. I was like a fish out of water. I looked to newly evolving scientific research for pieces of the puzzle to come together.

Spending hours pouring over libraries of scientific research wasn't the answer either. I had neither the time nor the energy. I had to focus on my priorities. Faith, trust and health came first. Everything else followed after that.

I sought out inspirational messages. Having learned early the value of emotions in healing, such things as fun, pleasure and joy were high priorities. It was natural for these to involve family, friends and church.

Eventually, there were long periods of time when my illness would improve. Then something like a flu epidemic would occur. I would catch the disease and when my resistance was down, this mysterious illness would be reactivated.

Over three years ago it happened again. This time the complications were worse than usual and getting well has been spasmodic. Although the healing feelings have been working and I have learned valuable new insights, it has been a very rocky road.

Throughout the process I have been convinced that the understandings to healings were in the real world. To me they had long ago been demystified. I did not claim to understand all healings because there are those accomplished through the laying on of hands or through prayer. Externally they are different. Internally, within the human body, the processes are basically the same.

Some people have developed their skills of healing hands. There are those of therapeutic touch used by some nurses and those of faith healing through the laying on of hands in various branches of Christianity. I have had enough experience in these other kinds of healing to realize they exist. Do I believe they are the result of Supreme Wisdom, God? Yes. I also think there are areas that have been studied and researched which will eventually explain them. Information on things like magnetic energy and mental telepathy has barely been tapped. What seems far-fetched today may be reality tomorrow, as we have often witnessed in recent decades. This is not only true in science and medicine but in religion as well.

The God in whom I believe does not play chess games with human lives nor does He play favorites. For one person to be healed while countless others ask for healing and are rejected, simply doesn't fit my understandings of God.

As I have been regaining my health, I have been writing. More of the pieces have been coming together. My material has been critiqued by doctors, pastors, fellow writers and friends. Notes or letters have been included in some of the chapters they have received. The following pages are from those letters. This may help explain my perspectives and experiences.

CHAPTER XIX

DEAR DOCTOR NO. 1

Dear Dr. Kalar,

Thanks for the tests and test results. It certainly requires a lot of doctor, patient trust. You are greatly appreciated.

I may not have been giving you a very clear picture of how I have been feeling. I have used terms like "gut level" and "deathly sick" but they could mean a lot of different things depending on who said them and how they were interpreted. Furthermore, it has occurred to me that whether the mind makes the body well or the patient is well, a person could look the same. This might be confusing.

My priorities muddle the issue because enthusiasm for healing exercises usually takes precedence over how I physically feel. While I have experienced most of these physical problems before, I am always learning something new about how to reverse or cope with them. Still, I keep asking myself, If I'm so good at mind exercises, why is it taking so long to feel better and have it hold?

One stumbling block is over-confidence. Because I'm always pushing for wellness, I latch on to signs of wellness and run with the ball when I should be walking. This has happened a couple times when I felt "normal" for several days only to end up back at base one. Still, it is a workable gage of my progress. I do know that spontaneous feelings of joy, adoration and praise (as opposed to intentional ones) need to be taken into account when evaluating a situation. They are easily overlooked.

It might be wise for me to reevaluate my expectations of wellness. You recall I quit taking a diuretic when this regimen of concentration exercises began early in 1995. They clearly caused frequent urination and diuretics were no longer necessary.

Some of the mind-body exercises have helped control my blood pressure. Others relax me. Most importantly, the healing feelings bring body chemistries back into balance.

I had been hoping to arrive at a point where I could forget these kinds of practices and go back to the "normal days". That may not be realistic. It may be wise to find a new and different perspective.

Not long ago, it occurred to me that the unique amount of mind-body exercises I use may require more minerals. Since we are talking about mechanisms and not something mystical, these greatly increased chemical activities could require more fuel. That might explain why I have needed extra minerals five times a day for three years. It has been necessary to trust my instincts to solve some of these problems.

Most insights I have received over the years have been as the result of looking back over what I have experienced, applying logic, and confirming it with what was acceptable medical, scientific or reasonable understandings.

If there are exceptions to the rule here, there are more than one. My years of dynamic mind techniques cannot be ignored. It's mind-body exercises that have brought body chemistries back into balance and prevented more serious complications from specific health problems time and again.

Few doctors have been aware of this. Most of them wouldn't have believed me if I'd told them. In fact I've been misused, abused, confused and sometimes amused by the reactions of medical people.

The mind-body techniques I use require more awareness of internal physical happenings. On the other hand I have a much greater objectivity than average. It has been essential, but it would have been difficult to achieve without my religious perspectives.

I suppose what is most significant to me is the way I have learned to influence the physical core of existence, the center of being. Certainly the central nervous system is at the heart of it all. Little wonder that I have had such strong religious convictions about understanding the center of being and the core of life.

Thanks,
Jean

CHAPTER XX

DEAR DOCTOR NO. 2

Dear Dr. Kalar,

I received additional material from Topeka regarding biofeedback. Since this came from offices that specialize in biofeedback, it has greater details. This is more like it!

I am always thrilled when respected authorities support the perspectives I've gained through forty years of experiences. This new material is exciting because much of it is like reading a review of the understandings I pieced together.

There is one main difference of emphasis. My views are as the result of religious experiences that led to the recognition of emotions in the link between mind and body health. Medical science usually rejects religious perspectives in this arena because there is the implication of dependence upon external forces. Clearly, that is a matter of insufficient understandings.

Although the mind-body connection has been well established, its acceptance has been relatively slow, even among mainstream medical people. The less informative brochure I received a few weeks ago is an example of that.

Interestingly, children learn mind controls more easily because they do not carry adult guilt, prejudices and fears. When I read about a boy with an inoperable brain tumor who learned to use biofeedback (and visualization) to influence his wellness, I was filled with joy.

Adults have some problems to overcome. Although decades of research have demonstrated that stress, anxiety and tension play a significant role in causing disease, it appears to be a mighty leap in the other direction to say the mind can make us well. Yet they are opposite extremes of the same mechanisms.

Instead of focusing on the controversy over positive and negative mind influences, it is useful to be aware of the greater perspectives. The new Topeka material led to the following statements.

1. Once we have learned mind control anywhere in our bodies, we have that power for life.

2. Skill at mind exercises helps to give the individual power over their life and health. At the same time it reduces weakness and dependency on outside controls.
3. Mind-body exercises are applicable to any kind of health problem.
4. Mind-body healing is not a miracle. It is use of mechanisms within our bodies that we each possess. This is how we were created. These are gifts we have each been given. Having recognized them, like many other mysteries of life and creation, we have the option to learn to use, enhance and develop them.
5.* Every change in the physical body is accompanied by a corresponding change in the mental, emotional condition. Likewise, every change in the mental, emotional state on conscious and subconscious levels brings about corresponding changes in the physical condition.
6. The body has intelligence in every cell that is constantly struggling to survive. We are already involved in this process every day and night on conscious and subconscious levels. We are not creating something new when we learn to amplify such processes. We are enhancing what already exists. The potential is open-ended.

It is valuable to learn that whenever a new neuropeptide is discovered, receptors are later found for these new peptides on immune system cells. This proves the immune system receives messages from the CNS. Amazingly, the immune system cells manufacture the same neuropeptides and send messages back to the CNS or central nervous system.

The same chemicals in the brain that control moods, perceptions and actions are also made by the immune system. The understandings of the circuit are complete.

Long ago I reasoned that anger was created by the mind and could cause the body to react, so why wouldn't dynamic religious feelings have a great impact upon the body? In my case it was obvious that they were healing.

This began my forty-year journey with "healing feelings".

Thanks,
Jean

* The psychophysiological principle affirms that, "Every change in the physiological state is accompanied by an appropriate change in the mental-emotional state, conscious or unconscious, and conversely, every change in the mental-emotional state, conscious or unconscious, is accompanied by an appropriate change in the physiological state."

Dr. Elmer E. Green

CHAPTER XXI

THE POWER OF BELIEVING

Faith is a word we easily relate to religion. While we can have faith in our parents, teachers or priests, most commonly faith seems to be expressed related to religion. The word, believing, by comparison seems to be much broader. We can believe in science, our team, fertilizer or a diet. Believing denotes a certain amount of trust but it does not expect infallibility. Faith, I think, leans more strongly toward perfection.

We can believe in irrational, illogical and unreasonable things. We can believe in things we cannot see, experience or feel. What is amazing about the whole scenario of believing is its power.

In the greater scheme of things, in the infinite picture, believing is a force for survival, both on the individual level and for the survival of the species in general. Faith and belief thoughts are recorded with higher priority in the brain. Therefore they play an important role in the mind-body chemistry and the survival of the individual.

Ironically, these mechanisms do not guarantee that our perspectives of belief are accurate. We can believe in things that are physically destructive, both externally and internally. We can believe in unhealthful nutrition, destructive forms of exercise, and practices, such as too much exposure to the sun, which can be dangerous to one's health.

Still, the fact that we have powerful mechanisms for faith and believing is not where the trouble lies. The problem lies in our lack of understandings. We make unwise choices because of ignorance.

When a person believes in demons, evil spirits or the devil, they may have the tendency to be aware of, or caught up in, negative perspectives. Truly believing in the actual existence of evil spirits goes beyond merely accepting the positive and negative experiences of life. This kind of thinking places such thoughts in higher priority in the brain and consequently they have a greater impact upon the mind and body.

That is why in civilizations where voodoo is practiced, people have been known to die because they believed they were cursed. This demonstrates the incredible power of the human mind. Yet it is interesting to note that people who do not believe in evil spirits are not affected by such demons.

Theologians sometimes point out that all creation is composed of positives and negatives, therefore, since there is a God, there must also be a devil.

We have finite vision regarding our God. Our roots teach us He is outside of, above, and beyond us on one hand. On the other hand He is within us, everywhere and constant. Biblical authors may have leaned toward the former teachings because those were within their comprehension. That perspective also made it easier to accept evil spirits with some rational.

Because we know there is precision in every atom and perfection in every cell, an infinitely greater perspective of God has been emerging. Much of what we have learned in twentieth century science has rocketed us to mental views far beyond anything known in past centuries.

Religious understandings evolve relative to what we comprehend about creation. In this era we understand the universe is billions of years old and for a significant portion of that time there was no life on earth. Through eons of time, life evolved from simple celled forms into higher creatures. We know that dinosaurs were part of that existence for millions of years.

Little wonder that we have difficulty fitting our Bible teachings about creation into what science tells us today. That does not mean science is wrong. Nor does it mean our faith has been misplaced.

The Bible is a collection of stories and teachings meant to illustrate, encourage and build faith. Faith can be more important than eating or sleeping. Faith can make the difference between life and death.

Sometimes humans have trouble recognizing that all of our learning is relative to Supreme Wisdom or God. We have difficulty realizing that religion is only part of our learning. Furthermore, we sometimes forget that creation doesn't exist because of religion but religion exists because of inquisitive human minds. Our thoughts, experiences and attempts to understand are the basis for religious teachings.

A form of faith on subconscious levels has helped us to live, evolve and survive. Perhaps, this is more closely related to what we know as instinct. As human beings we see this in other creatures of nature but we have a tendency to think of ourselves as above or outside of this natural process of wisdom in creation.

Science seems to tell us the purpose of life is life. In other words faith is built into the processes of life.

For decades science has revealed how the defense mechanisms of the body are constantly fighting bacteria, viruses, fungi, molds, etc. Electron microscopes disclosed far more viruses and other foreign matter battling in this endless war than we had ever imagined.

We know respiration, circulation and digestion are vital life forces. We have not been so quick to add all human thoughts and actions. It's true, we accept certain constructive, intelligent actions as life preserving. It is more difficult to see beyond those.

While faith on subconscious levels helped us to live, evolve and survive, when we became more highly developed our conscious mind added many complications to this picture. If we had remained primitive we would have relied on our instincts and inherited survival skills. Once we evolved past that phase we had feelings and questions which opened broader vistas. On one hand this was positive. On the other hand it was complicating and confusing.

To feel in awe of a rainbow, a sunset or a butterfly caused thinking man to experience special emotions. At first there were questions of how and why.

Reasoning humans, in the absence of knowledge of billions of years of evolution and multi-trillions or more of evolutionary processes, assumed these things were planned by someone far superior and greater than we. Because humans could design and create, we assumed this was also true of nature. We could build houses, weapons and things of beauty. Surely the incredible facets of nature were designed by someone too. But it would need to be an infinitely greater Creator than man.

There were feelings on one hand of wonder, awe and appreciation. This caused concepts of inferiority and guilt. But more than this, through it all, there were feelings of being connected with a Higher Power, Creator or God.

Biblical authors could not have known that through all those eons of evolution the body processes that were incorporated into each human being for survival were being formed and recorded in our genes. They could not have known that the emotions of love, joy and faith were among the facets of survival recorded in our bodies.

Because of the endless ways in which faith can enrich our lives, the Bible was written. Critics would say there is no logic to many of its teachings.

For instance, how could Noah, who was in Africa, have had polar bears, elk or reindeer from North America on his boat? How could he have carried kangaroos and koala bears from Australia and thousands of other creatures unknown to Africa on his ark?

The question of the virgin birth usually arouses the ire of critics of the Bible. And there are many more.

We do not need to believe the literal interpretations of all Bible stories to understand the value of faith and what faith did for our forefathers. Faith is just as valuable today as it has always been.

In fact, faith is more valuable today than it was for our forefathers. Today we can better grasp the reality of how our thoughts affect body chemistry, our lives and survival.

Where healing is concerned, we know the mind influences body chemistry through constant emotional interpretations of thoughts and experiences. This is done on subconscious levels. What is even more significant is the fact that healing can be enhanced and its essential chemistries dramatically multiplied through conscious practices that direct the bodies healing forces. With the addition of greater understandings and stronger beliefs, the body's capacity to produce more healing chemistry is enriched still further.

The possibilities of the power of believing are limited only by each individual.

CHAPTER XXII

THE RIVER OF LIFE

Seen as God sees them all things are alive and beautiful.
                                                        ... Henry David Thoreau

Many times I have questioned if I could be so keenly tuned in to the core of life that I have consciously manipulated, changed or enriched life's healing forces. Since I have proven these processes countless times, I inevitably arrive at the same conclusion. Yes.

Why have I been allowed to have this corner of understandings on the secrets of life? When I feel unworthy my question is more along the lines of "Why me?".

Then I rationalize and tell myself it's no big deal. Everyone has healing mechanisms. Our bodies subconsciously use them all the time for the processes of life. Amazingly religious people have unknowingly or mysteriously manipulated them for centuries. Besides, mind-body enhancement such as biofeedback has been practiced in the medical community for more than three decades. These mechanisms are all related.

We are in an era where we can comprehend that human beings all over the world have similar body chemistry, common mechanisms and equal potential for disease reversals. Although these things occur on different levels and in a wide variety of ways, what is most important is the recognition of their existence and their innate worth.

Of course God is the source of such healings. It is supreme Wisdom that caused such body processes to come into existence. This is the way we were created. These are our gifts.

The fact that faith healings evolved through religion is logical because it is in religion that the feelings are greater and more noticeable. From my experience they stimulate, enhance and enrich the core healing mechanisms of life.

Nature knew this. Humans did not. That did not stop evolution from building upon these kinds of things. Mankind does not exist outside of the laws and principles of nature. In fact we are dependent upon them. We cannot survive without them.

Supreme Wisdom, God, exists in these principles just as God exists everywhere in creation. Our greatest difficulty is in filling the black holes of our ignorance.

Much of our faith is limited by our understandings. Furthermore, we find it difficult to make adjustments in our beliefs because it becomes threatening. What we believe is part of who we are. That is why these kinds of changes do not come easily.

In the beginning I recognized sensations. In the beginning my focus was on noticing how the different feelings were experienced. I soon learned healing sensations were related to religious passions of awe, adoration, love and joy.

It didn't occur to me that it might seem sacrilegious to analyze religious feelings. Most Christians believed such sensations came from God, the Holy Spirit, or Jesus. Most people believed they were of something other than the real world. That's why they were considered to be holy or divine.

My perspective insisted there were no miracles in "God's eyes". To God all things were known and real. This meant there were understandings and answers available. We were the ones who needed to find the answers and solve the mysteries.

Initially, I did not set out to find solutions any more than I set out to be healed. It was spontaneous, natural religious experiences that caused feelings of wellness for me. When I realized nothing new had entered my body, I was forced to make a major turnaround in my mental view.

Understandings of faith healings were of such value to mankind that I felt drawn to the Bible and its prophecies. I found a reference to such an event in Revelation where a "pure river of water of life" is described. But since much of the book of Revelation is written in unclear symbolism, I could hardly claim its descriptions as proof of anything.

Yet, to have discovered, consciously used and received healing energy from mechanisms within my own body could not have been more beautifully described than with words like the "pure river of water of life".

The subconscious mind, I am convinced, is involved in all of our mind-body processes. It is involved in all of our health, healing and survival. Some people might say the subconscious mind can be destructive. Yet all life constantly struggles to survive. Therefore, the subconscious mechanisms are not the problem. It is our limited knowledge concerning them that presents difficulties.

Whether we see the subconscious mind at work in psychosomatic illnesses or stigmata, we think of them as isolated incidents in which the mind influences the body. This is not true. The mind is constantly influencing body chemistry... always striving for survival of the individual or survival of the species in general.

In that domain are vast complications.

CHAPTER XXIII

PRINCIPLES AND PERSPECTIVES

My people are destroyed from lack of knowledge:
Hosea 4:6

For thousands of years our forefathers have known the value of faith and the belief in a Higher Power. Mystery and mysticism became interwoven and intertwined with their ancient beliefs and they remained a significant part of the evolution of understandings.

The Bible is full of stories of incredible faith. Critics would have to acknowledge that there are life saving, life changing, even the saving of whole clans of people through acts of faith in this holy book. A person might question the wisdom of some decisions made by Biblical characters but greater examples of human faith are hard to find. Sometimes the stories seem to have been enhanced or glorified in the Bible, but the reader needs to remember the beliefs of Biblical authors were less sophisticated than ours. They wrote and acted according to understandings of their times.

Not only was this true thousands of years ago, but it has been true in the centuries that followed. As a result, the unfolding of new insights and understandings has been relatively slow. Yet, Protestantism and its many branches have evolved through a new awareness and discernment as the result of inspired leaders.

Building faith has always been man's main concern in this arena. However, faith was not always recognized as their primary goal. It may have been confused in issues of national pride, demons, war or lust. Still, if one is logical, the greatest value of religion has been that of building faith.

While concepts of angels, heavenly rewards and favors enriched beliefs, teachings of punishment, destruction and hell were meant to counter the "evil", doubtful or less enthusiastic worshippers.

Depending upon individual personalities and what they have been taught, different aspects of prophesied End Times have been important in relative ways. For years there were those who were eager for their rewards and the punishment of the ungodly.

At the same time a view of God was emerging which saw Him as all loving, ever present, all knowing, understanding and forgiving. Built upon the foundations of Christian faith preserved by our forefathers, this broader and brighter view of God has emphasized scriptures often denied or misunderstood in the past.

Our humanness exudes in teachings of punishments, rewards and revenge. For centuries we built our faith upon these concepts. They were meant to bring control over human actions when there were no better answers.

There are few areas of Christianity where less agreement exists than in the End Time predictions. Some prefer to ignore them altogether. Others stay away from them because of fear. Still others have painstakingly related the animals and tribulations in Revelation to countries, wars and catastrophes of nature in this era. More than once a group of sincere believers has gathered in some remote mountain convinced that the end of the world was at hand.

There are descriptions of veils being lifted, the heavens opening up and people no longer seeing as through a dark glass. All of these words define seeing or understanding through the revelation of truths. If there is one thing most believers could agree upon, it is the need for understandings.

To understand centuries of religious mysteries could not be more appropriately described than "and they need no candle, neither light of the sun; for the Lord God giveth them light:" Revelation 22: 5. Knowing truths about life and death, heaven and hell, suffering and sorrow, rewards and punishments, are interests of most concerned Christians.

Numerous hymns have repeatedly verbalized these concerns. Religious music is one of the best expressions of the depth of our feelings and the longings of our hearts. This does not mean hymns repeat truths or facts. Great music, however, touches our hearts in ways only music can do. Hymns about streets of gold and choirs of angels embrace the mysteries and joys of our faith but they are still mysteries.

We may say we want answers but do we? Sometimes I wonder whether we wouldn't rather savor the mystery and miracles of religion so that the concepts upon which our faith has been founded need not be changed. Changing religious beliefs does not come easily.

Still, understandings come in the real world. They come in terms we can comprehend. Isn't that what revelations are all about?

CHAPTER XXIV

LIFTING VEILS

Nature never did betray the heart that loved her.
...William Wordsworth

Recently, national news proclaimed that human beings are "wired for God". The media was saying that California scientists have found the "God Module" in the brain. In other words, with machines that test human brains, researchers could identify the area where people emotionally and psychologically experience God.

These tests were done with people who have an unusual kind of epilepsy. Intense religious and mystical experiences are common for them. The fact that a specific kind of epileptic has made it possible for scientists to identify what part of the brain religious experiences occur means it is very likely the area is the same for the rest of us. After all, epileptics have difficulty with neurological impulses, not with their thinking.

Countless religious people may have dismissed this study of California researchers with little thought. However, there is a much deeper meaning worth exploring. When St. Augustine said our souls cannot rest until we have found God, it is now more than a theological theory.

In highly specific tests, scientists learned that the brain involuntarily responded stronger to religious words as the result of the patient's seizures. The researchers theorized that these dedicated and ancient processes of the brain may have evolved to strengthen ties of friends and family or build tribal loyalty.

What researchers may have missed is the healing value the emotional interpretation of these religious experiences brings. As the body constantly strives for wellness, it performs life saving feats on all levels. While it is known that all thoughts are emotionally interpreted and endorphins (among many other body chemistries) are produced as the result of religious experiences, we do not know the exact role such chemistries play in stopping, controlling or reversing these epileptic seizures.

It is significant that religious thoughts and experiences are not merely whimsical happenings or surface decisions. St. Augustine could have more appropriately said, "We are wired for God". The temporal lobe of the brain shows we are wired for religious experiences.

Religion and science have had their disagreements but this discovery narrows the gap. It recognizes the credibility of religion without getting involved in the truths and falsehoods in this arena. The religious experience is real. It is our translations that have been somewhat diverse.

With perfection in every atom and intelligence in every cell we can be assured that there is a reason and purpose for all things. Except where interference occurs, life is constantly fulfilling its preprogrammed design of survival. There is little question that the area of the brain "wired" for religious experiences is part of that survival. The emotional interpretations that take place as the result of that area of the brain and how they affect our body chemistry is a great breakthrough.

And so we come full circle. Religiously we have always proclaimed the value of faith. We have taught, nurtured and protected the significance of our beliefs. On conscious levels faith, the top priority of religion, has strengthened us through pain, suffering and sorrow. Faith, believing in Supreme Wisdom, a Higher Power, or God, has not been a figment of our imaginations. Our concepts of God have been part of our very existence, recorded in the depths of our being.

We have struggled to put our beliefs into words. We have interpreted them in many different religions and faiths. Still, in spite of our diversity, some things come through loud and clear. We are created to have faith, think about and feel connected to a Higher Power, God.

It was countless evolutionary forces that led to the forces of human life and their chemistries for survival. These were recorded in our brains with high priority and the body chemistries connected with them have been for our survival.

Modern science can name many of these chemicals. One of them is serotonin that became a part of life early in the evolutionary processes. Serotonin is a substance that is important in mood, pain, sleep, appetite and countless essential feelings.

A variety of drugs used to treat depression, obesity, and things like migraine headache are known to act upon the serotonin mechanisms. Serotonin is intrinsic to an amazing part of the body known as the enteric system. These nerves stretch from the neck to the colon and they are where numerous "gut feelings" are created. Many things once thought to be "in the head" are now known to be involved with these mechanisms.

At least 100 million nerve cells in the "gut" act as a "second brain" and are constantly communicating with the brain. Little wonder that we have religiously described a river of feelings that flow from deep within our being. Until recently we believed that all emotional feelings originated in the head.   We now know these things are much more complicated. Mysteries are becoming understandings.

Serotonin was an essential part of the early life processes.   It was a major factor in building the core mechanisms for survival.   Serotonin cannot be ignored as a significant part of a religious experience or a healing.

When we describe feelings such as God in our soul, love of Jesus in our heart, or the Holy Spirit in the depths of our being, the enteric nerves are the most likely mechanisms to be affected. Little wonder that emotions of joy, adoration, and love are involved in the production of serotonin and the body's healing chemistries.

MY PRAYER

Oh God, if I could lay my hands
On folks and make them well,
I would give more praise to thee
Then words could ever tell.

My child wait just a little while
I have a better plan.
The era is upon us now
When folks will understand.
Then healings will be common place
In folks throughout the land.

Jean A. Pentico

CHAPTER XXV

DEAR DOCTOR NO. 3

Dear Dr. Kalar,

I was pretty sure I had explained my corner of understandings quite well. There are scientific facts to support my experiences and personal views on faith healings, disease reversals:

1. The life force = emotions.
2. The healing feelings = passions and religious feelings.
3. The core of life = emotional feelings and their interactions with essential body mechanisms.
4. Disease reversals and faith healings are the same mechanisms.
5. Positive emotions are involved in health and healing in subconscious ways on a daily basis.
6. Disease reversals are a greater relative form of the same emotional mechanisms in number five, above.
7. Intense positive emotions and passions are a dynamic part of disease reversals, faith healings.

Still, as you've noticed, I haven't had great luck making these healing processes "hold" with this chronic illness. There have been a number of unanswered questions.

A review of Christian denominations that focus on faith healings and reject medical help reveals an important principle. They insist that a person needs to totally, invincibly believe they are healed.

Obviously I do better when I have understandings. The "healing feelings" I understand quite well. But what are the processes necessary to make them hold for this health problem? They have worked for other healing needs. What has been missing here?

In "Molecules of Emotion" Dr. Candace B. Pert describes emotions at the molecular level of peptides and peptide receivers. The mind and body are constantly communicating at the cellular level. Often the same chemistries are manufactured in the body, which were once assumed to come only from the brain. More importantly, this communication is due to the chemistries of emotion. In other words body cells have specific receptors for emotion. The essential role of emotions in human life and survival is confirmed and clarified.

Bodymind is a term used in recent years and one that Dr. Pert embraces. The oneness of the body and mind is not easy to grasp because most of us grew up recognizing the mind and body as separate but connected entities.

In "Alphabet of the Heart" Dan Winter suggests that the resonant location of emotions on the double helix determines the location of active or inactive genetic codes. Resonance translates to vibrations. Dr. Pert also refers to vibrations at the molecular level. The vibrations of different facets of life and creation are a part of us that for the most part are not experienced on a conscious level. Yet vibrations play an important role in how the DNA is formed.

Dr. Candace B. Pert, as a young graduate student, laid the foundation for the discovery of endorphins. As a former chief of brain biochemistry she worked at the National institutes of Health for thirteen years.

Dr. Pert was involved with research when it was found that the nervous system, endocrine and immune systems function integratedly. This led to the new field of psychoneuroimmunology.

It has long been known that about sixty percent of the genetic code has blank frames. This has been a puzzling phenomenon. Researchers now believe that blank frames allow for bodily adaptations according to our survival needs. In fact there is some evidence of this happening in HIV patients as well as cancer and other health survival studies. It is happening within individual lifetimes. These are considered to be spontaneous but the role of emotions cannot be ignored.

In the past we assumed it took generations for genetic codes to be formed. Still, for some time there have been hints that such understandings were incomplete.

When Dr. Weil suggested that passions of love could activate latent genes and cause disease reversals, he was probably on target. But what makes the difference between a temporary and a permanent healing?

Amazingly, there appears to be truth in what the faith healing experts have been saying all these years. In fact the truth is rooted in what Christ said when he proclaimed that faith is what makes one whole or well.

Belief mechanisms seem to be part of the answer to making a healing hold. Studies show that emotion combined with logic or beliefs make the difference. If something is logical, we believe it. For most people who have been healed through their religion, faith has been their logic. Emotion has been a sideline not always noticed or appreciated. In fact because of social stigmas connected with emotion, such feelings may have even been denied.

Scientists have been very careful to point out that it is more than thoughts. We can't simply think away illnesses.

Thoughts are an essential part of the picture. Emotions are also vital. But it appears to be belief or logic that is necessary to change DNA.

Since 1995 valuable research has been done in this area. Stanford University, the Institute of HeartMath, the University of Alabama and AIDS research centers were involved in vital studies which led to understandings of spontaneous disease reversals in patients with HIV, cancer, etc. They found emotion combined with logic caused healing changes in DNA.

These researchers were coming from different perspectives than I. Still, the common denominators were there. Belief systems equal religious persuasions. The pieces fit. At the same time both religious and non-religious healings can be explained.

Writing this in black and white makes it sound cold and far too easy to achieve healing. You know how hard I've worked to get well and stay that way. In spite of the struggles, I have embraced life. I have danced the dance. You know this material is the result of my firsthand knowledge of its worth.

One question haunts me, though, would it have been easier if I hadn't wanted to *explain* what my heart knows to be true?

THANKS,
Jean

CHAPTER XXVI

WHAT IS REAL?

Would the understandings given to me be more convincing if I had been diagnosed with something critical, such as cancer, and had overcome it through the principles described in these pages? Whenever I'm faced with a question like that I look for the greater answer. We have a tendency to put God in a box or, in other words, restrict the scope of God. Therefore in seeking religious answers it is often useful to look beyond what we have always accepted. How can folks benefit the most? What is the greater intent?

We have heard of miraculous healings. Relative to what is needed, there are mighty few. Another miracle would hardly make us better informed. Neither would there be any way to answer all of the questions about the quality of the cancer diagnosis, the errors in laboratory work or any other doubts folks could imagine.

What would be for the greater good of mankind? It is not enough to say I have survived forty years because of the use of these principles. Nor would it be helpful to refer to the many times my potentially serious and even critical illnesses have been reversed through these practices. All of that could be questioned and pronounced unprovable.

What is likely to be most helpful? It appears that a fresh understanding on how we can consciously influence the principles of life for healing would be good. If we can comprehend the logical mechanisms at work in using the mind to multiply life's healing processes, we have made a giant step. That way any person desiring to overcome their illness could apply such principles and have chances to reverse their own health problem with the support and help of the medical profession. This is what I have attempted to explain.

One major problem is how we view health and our own responsibility in wellness. In a way, our society teaches us to expect someone else to help us. There is no doubt we can glean much help from other professionals and experts, but we need a better understanding of the value of what we can do and how powerful our mind is in the healing process. We know the value of exercise. We learn more every day about hidden nutrients in fruits, vegetables and the foods we eat that go far beyond vitamins and minerals.

When this information is placed in our hands, we can make better choices. We have been given greater control over our life and health.

When it comes to disease, we have the right to make wiser choices and be actively involved in getting well. If the understandings of life are beyond our range of knowledge we can find ourselves at the mercy of ignorance.

We know physical exercise, nutrition, and faith are valuable. How many of us have explored meditation and other forms of stress-relieving exercises to enhance our health? It may be necessary to take nutritional supplements on a regular basis. A person can learn about herbs and alternative medicines that apply to their health problem. There are books on wellness written for lay people. Taking a determined and active role in one's own health can make a surprising difference.

However, once we have recognized the vital role emotions play in health, healing and life's processes, we have made a quantum leap in our understandings of survival. It is clear that belief systems need to precede emotions because beliefs will determine whether emotions are positive or negative. Even so, emotions are the key.

CHAPTER XXVII

THE QUANTUM LEAP

Once we recognize the vital role emotions play in human wellness, we can see the proof of emotions at work in all forms of life. We have always been surrounded by sensory stimulation. We have evolved, developed and survived dependant upon how our senses have responded to it all. Not only have humans, the highest of the evolutionary scale, developed through these processes, all other forms of life have evolved relative to these principles for millions of years. We are related to all forms of life in these developments. We are at one with Creation, Supreme Wisdom, God in these forces.

While most of this information has been known for ages, we still have a tendency to see ourselves in a modern society barely related to those eons of evolution. We prefer to think we are something outside of all other forms of life. Yet it is in recognizing how we are "put together" that we become aware of how we can survive some of life's most critical ills. While the sensory role in the development of life on our planet has long been recognized, the newest aspect of the survival of life is in recognizing the vital role emotions play in this drama.

Many of us have assumed only humans have valuable emotions and that they were nonessential. Thanks to Public Television, The Learning Channel, The Discovery Channel, etc., millions of people have learned about emotions of the many species of animals. Dog lovers, who have long insisted their pets smiled when they were happy, could see the true evidence. Pictures of sorrowing chimpanzees who had lost a baby were shown. Elephants could be seen displaying incredible concern and tenderness for their young, sharing in the care of each other's babies and going to amazing extremes to save a baby fallen in a mud hole. In finding an elephant's dead skeleton, they appeared to be disturbed as they paced around the bones.

Wolves, the forefathers of dogs, reveal roles within the pack, which show expressions of emotion relative to their rank. Some actions insist upon supremacy, and emotional feelings are obvious as these animals react to other members of their wolf pack.

The evidence for such feelings in animals, birds and insects has been described in countless ways by those who specialize in such studies. As humans we may have seen these things as interesting aspects of animal life but we have been slow to recognize how vital emotions have been in the development and survival of each life form. We have maintained that emotions were frosting on the cake of life. We didn't realize emotions were truly the nuts and bolts of our existence.

There have been more than hundreds of billions of life processes at work in creating life and helping each specie develop their own survival mechanisms. The basic rule in nature seems to have been, "If it feels good, it enhances life". From the most simple forms of life, such as the amoeba, to the most complicated human beings, every developmental process of digestion, respiration, skin color, bone structure, intelligence and more, have evolved relative to emotional interpretations. Those things that "felt good" and enhanced life were retained. Obviously, those things which led to the destruction of life were eventually left behind.

When we think of how some creatures are drawn to sunlight and others prefer darkness, we know this is the result of their sensory perceptions and the emotional interpretations they have made. Bats and certain insects can hear hundreds of times better than humans, relative to their emotional feelings and their needs to survive. Dogs and most wild animals have a sense of smell far superior to humans. Again, this evolved relative to their survival. Some creatures can see in all directions depending upon which way they turn their eyes. Some flying birds can see a mouse running on the ground at heights beyond anything humans could imagine.

Not only is emotion at the basis of all these developments, as you can see, it is at the core of existence. We have a kinship with all forms of life because of this survival principle. Not only is it seen in creatures, it is recognized in the more primitive forms such as plant life.

Sensitivity systems in plants, trees, flowers and grasses help them grow toward the sun, spread roots to reach for water and react to a variety of stimulants which they interpret in some primitive emotional way as good or bad for their endurance. This is more evident in parts of the country where there are four seasons and plants respond to these changes. Then trees lose their leaves in the fall and spring brings forth buds and new growth according to stimulants.

Not many years ago studies were done with houseplants which indicated they responded to loving care, music and other aspects of human life we thought were absurd. Yet the more we recognize there are sensitivity systems in all forms of life which have enabled us to persist, the more we become aware of a dimension in creation we have greatly ignored. The value in all this is that of recognizing what makes us "tick" and the priority life places on emotions.

The human brain has 100 billion neurons which are involved with how our emotions affect our cells. Such quantities we have trouble comprehending. Researchers tell us these mechanisms far exceed the finest computer. Little wonder that we have difficulty, from a religious point of view, grasping the myriads of processes essential in the development of human life. Little wonder we have not seen the vital role emotions play in our healing.

CHAPTER XXVIII

THE "FEEL GOOD" DILEMMA

Since it is built into the systems of life to seek "feel good" things, it should be no surprise when this becomes a major problem in our society. Feeling good can be at the basis of greed, corruption, addictions, crime and more. Such behavior can be destructive to other humans, animals and our environment. The "feel good" principle is very primitive and preceded logic or intelligence in our evolutionary development.

For millions of years nature has built these basic urges into our very mechanisms because, for the most part, they have worked quite well in our survival. This principle has been very successful in primitive creatures. Wild animals usually kill only what they can eat, take care of their own and respect each other's territories. In general, wild creatures find pleasure in hunting, eating, sleeping, grooming and other acts of life that they control and need. The majority of wild creatures have something or some other creature to fear but animals act and react. They may become anxious but worry is more evident in humans. Because of intelligence we have the capacity to find many more reasons to worry.

Intelligence gives us vastly increased resources for survival. It also adds dimensions to life that can bring destruction. If we didn't understand so much we wouldn't get into trouble so often. We wouldn't find ourselves persuaded to indulge in destructive behavior by those who are our peers or leaders. Drugs, incest, rape and pedophilia are part of this picture. While it is frustrating and discouraging to have outside influences mislead us, we often become our own worst enemies when it comes to addiction.

In addiction, eons of evolution tell us it feels good so it must be good for us. These very basic, primitive urges, which have proven their worth throughout the ages, turn into destructive actions. Logically, intelligence should take over and draw appropriate boundaries. Clearly, this is not always so. Alcohol, drugs and smoking can become addictive and harmful for a number of reasons. These habits are not essential for the survival of life so one wonders why they can become such tragic forces. Personalities and genes become involved and these are very complicated factors.

Food addiction is a tricky one. Food, after all, is essential to life. For it to become a destructive force is bizarre. Again, intelligence should help us make wise choices. On the other hand, the pleasure principle combines with food, the earliest need for survival, and it becomes a double problem.

Then a third instinctive factor becomes involved. Stress, anxiety and tension need to be counterbalanced with pleasure. Our conscious mind may be telling us one thing while our age-old control mechanisms are repeatedly calling for something else.

Intelligent choices become mixed with personalities, stress, anxiety, tensions, and backgrounds. The whole picture explodes. Smuggling drugs, crime and other illegal acts involve personalities who may have believed these things would bring them good feelings. Human personalities can cause conduct to be distorted and twisted.

Even these explanations are an over simplification of complicated issues. Some habits, addictions and health problems are influenced by our genes and generations of difficulties with body chemistries.

The feel good principle is easier to identify in nature's more primitive creatures. Nevertheless, we are all part of the process. We wouldn't want it to be any other way.

LIFE'S LESSONS

Of all life's lessons
I have learned,
The one that I have truly earned
Is having faith.

Of all that I've been taught and heard
The wisdom of the written word
Is meaningless
Without experience that counts,
When one is tried in vast amounts,
And overcomes.

It's faith that triumphs over all
And makes each agonizing fall
A building block.
So I am glad that I am me
For faith has helped me to be free,
And I thank God!

Jean A. Pentico

CHAPTER XXIX

PARALLELS OF PASSION

Books on chakras have always seemed too mysterious for me. Lately I have broadened my perspective. For one thing, the mind-body exercises I have practiced all these years are related to what the Far East mediators have done for centuries. Furthermore, their mystical, spiritual view of emotions has evidently paralleled those of Western medicine for ages. After all it wasn't until recent decades that numerous emotions became body mechanisms with chemistries known to us.

Our newer scientific methods of analyzing emotions are different from the ancient techniques of the Far East. However, their approaches were not unlike mine in my quest to understand the healing chemistry in the body as the result of religious experiences.

There's an important chakra in the middle of the body that is called the "center of subconscious" or "first consciousness". I don't know how they arrived at this perspective but I do know the feelings in that location have always been of highest importance in my "healing feeling" concentrations. I learned the value of this location long ago because it is grounded in my original religious feelings.

Most of the mantras cause sensations much like those I experience in the center of the body. The vocal sounds of Aum and God are very similar. Obviously their vibrations would be related. Whole schools of thought are based upon the value of sound therapy for enriching health and healing. Just as specific sounds can shatter glass, it is believed that certain sounds can influence the flow of energy in the body. We need only to think of our favorite music or the songs of birds to recognize how positive the effects of sound can be. Normally we think it is the pleasing tones that influence us, yet at the mechanical level these things are heard because of vibrations.

Interestingly the Aum mantra is the crown mantra. It is on top of the head and connects a person to their Divine Source or Higher Power. These concepts parallel some of my religious views as well as countless others in the Western world.

By today's scientific understandings we know there is a "God Module" in the brain. This means there are areas of the brain that show specific activity during religious experiences. These can be recorded with some of the latest scientific equipment. Since all thoughts are emotionally interpreted and produce chemistry which affect the body, we automatically know words like Aum and God influence body chemistry.

It seems reasonable to consider that the first consciousness chakra or the subconscious chakra could be involved with the early development of man. In this location some of the earliest processes of evolution might well be recorded. This could explain the core of life information that can be healing and appears to be related to the center of the body in a religious experience.

Approaching this concept from a different angle, the solar plexus is in the center of the body. For centuries the solar plexus was believed to be the most vital part of life. A network of nerves forming our "second brain" lies here. By concentrating on the subconscious chakra and expanding it to a large ball, the solar plexus is easily included. This is an exercise highly recommended by chakra experts. Why? Is it because of feelings vital to life?

Just as the reptilian brain in humans recorded the early evolutionary processes of life, it appears that the solar plexus is the corresponding part of the body where sensations and feelings for survival developed. This compares to the first consciousness chakra and its correlating area in the brain. There is little doubt that some kind of brain/body connection was present in the earliest forms of evolving life. Some relative form exists in even the most primitive creatures. Always they embody the secrets of life and survival. Instinctively we have known this in a "spiritual" way. The God Module of the brain connects us with millions of years of creation, the Wisdom of the Ages, Universal Intelligence, our Higher Power. It is likely that it connects us with the subconscious chakra, the first consciousness chakra and the core mechanisms of life. These kinds of things can be involved in a healing experience.

Medical specialists who have studied spontaneous disease reversals, miracle cures and unexplained healings basically agree that personalities play a vital role. The famous alternative medicine doctor, Dr. Andrew Weil, says the intensity of emotional feelings is important. He encourages people to develop a passion. Healings have been known to occur when people fall in love or have some other great passion. He claims apathy may be the greatest deterrent to spontaneous healings.

I do not know how yogis of the Far East arrived at first consciousness chakras or the subconscious chakra. I can only surmise it was through feelings and using logic to try and identify or explain them. These kinds of techniques I could understand.

MORE OF LIFE'S LESSONS

We have billions of forces
Striving for our survival.
Some pull together.
Others seem like rivals.
Inside every atom,
Living creature and flower,
Perfection exists
Every day and each hour.
When life seems crazy
And we don't understand,
We know there's wisdom
On life's every hand.
We know there's perfection,
We can't comprehend
And we're being gifted
From now till life's end.
So it's faith that upholds us
And gives us strength when we're lost.
Then cling to your faith
Whatever the cost.

Jean A. Pentico

CHAPTER XXX

THE CORE OF LIFE

We know "gut feelings" are experienced in the middle of the body. Laughter is easily felt there. Norman Cousins helped us recognize the core of life processes that are enhanced through laughter. He became famous for reversing a potentially fatal disease by using laughter as a vital part of his regimen.

If laughter can reverse disease because of the core of life information in the "gut", why wouldn't special religious feelings reverse disease because of sensations in this area?

For years scientists have known there are 64 possible combinations for our genetic code. Yet only 20 are turned on. Why? Does this allow for disease reversals? We know survival information is encoded in every cell of our body.

Most of us think of the body and mind as separate entities. Dr. Candace Pert became famous for her research in how the mind affects the body. She coined the word, bodymind. The body and mind are so interconnected and interrelated that they cannot be separated. This is important to remember when we consider healings.

We can assume enzymes would be an essential part of a faith healing since they are highly specific and can be created by our body. They could dissolve the parts of cells that need correction and help bring about needed changes.

The emotional mechanisms, the limbic system, produce vast amounts of peptides, nueropeptides and polynutrients for the countless receptors in the body. Emotions have a powerful effect on the autonomic nervous system that regulates everything from how much insulin is secreted to defining our blood pressure levels. Emotions help the autonomic nervous system and the immune system communicate. The immune system has receptors for chemicals because of life-saving emotion.

It was Dr. Robert Ader, a psychologist who discovered the immune system, like the brain, can learn. Researchers tell us our body overcomes cancer many times in each life without our knowledge. The mechanisms for healing are gifts already given to us. Can we consciously influence them with our mind and emotions? Science says we not only can but we do. Reversing a serious illness, once it is established, may not be easy. Evidently we have the equipment to make it happen. What has been lacking is solid reason to believe this is true. Belief or faith based upon logic and reason can be more powerful than faith in miracles. Or can it? Would we have the passion to make healings happen? There is another important parallel between Far East meditations and what I have found most helpful in healing practices. The ball rolling up my spine and out the top of my head, mentioned earlier in this book, was a concept taken from a branch of Christianity where some of the Far East meditations were used. This ball of energy is compared to Kundalini, a vital part of chakra, mind-body exercises. I learned how to use the ball of energy in connection with "healing feelings" more than thirty years ago. At that time I knew nothing about chakras and emotions. In fact thirty years ago the related field of psychonueroimmunology was unknown.

Needless to say, I see mind-body biofeedback exercises playing a greater role in the future of medicine. While doctors diagnose, treat, test and support us in the processes of health, we can choose to accept a greater role in our healing and survival.

CHAPTER XXXI

EPILOGUE

It was my intent to share with you my experiences, beliefs and understandings. I felt sure that physical answers could be found to explain how some faith healings take place. I knew our emotions were involved. Clearly, faith and thoughts played a vital role. It did not occur to me that all thoughts were emotionally interpreted. I did not expect to find receptors are located all over the body that are involved in accepting the chemicals of emotion. These chemicals affect the immune system as well as disease reversals.

We know faith healings change cells, genes and sicknesses. Medically, biofeedback has been used to alter pain and disease. Now we are learning these healing processes are related. Religiously, we believe it's our faith in God that makes the difference. In medical science "belief systems" are identified as having a vital role, Obviously, belief systems and faith are closely related. The same mind-body mechanisms are at work. Various degrees of bodily healing can result.

The miracle of faith healings has long been mystical. Now it appears there are sufficient understandings to describe how emotions are essential in most of these changes. I didn't expect to recognize that all life is dependent upon sensations and some kind of emotional interpretation of them. For millions of years the evolution of each specie followed these basic pathways. Emotions have been intrinsically involved in the development of genes that make up life patterns.

We know emotions have the ability to affect the immune system. Furthermore, if these feelings have always been vital in the development of life's genes, why wouldn't they have the capacity to turn on inactive codes of DNA for faith healings?

Years ago I learned we can dramatically enhance our healing processes through faith and emotion. Science has come a long way in clarifying this. By understanding how these healing techniques work, we have solid ground for belief in faith healings.

Of course, there still are the healings through prayer or laying on of hands. Externally they may be different, but the same body mechanisms for healing are at work inside each one of us. The gifts have already been given.

Scientists have been limited in their efforts to study faith healings. Such disease reversals are relatively rare. Still, from a variety of sources there has been enough research to supply the understandings we need. I could not have known so much information would be available to explain my experiences and beliefs.

"Each patient carries his own doctor inside him. They come to us not knowing the truth. We are at our best when we give the doctor who resides within each patient a change to go to work."

...Albert Schweitzer

BIBLIOGRAPHY

Siegel, Bernie S., M.D.
LOVE MEDICINE AND MIRACLES
New York: Harper and Row, 1986

Simonton, 0. Carl, M.D.
Simonton, Stephanie Matthews
Creighton, James L.
GETTING WELL AGAIN
New York: Bantam Books, 1992

Chopra, Deepak, M.D.
QUANTUM HEALING
New York: Bantam Books, 1990

Weil, Andrew, M.D.
SPONTANEOUS HEALING
New York: Knopf, 1995

Dossey, Larry, M.D.
HEALING WORDS
New York: Harper Collins, 1993

Goleman, Daniel
EMOTIONAL INTELLIGENCE
New York: Bantam Books, 1995

Benson, Herbert, M.D.
THE RELAXATION RESPONSE
New York: Avon Books, 1976

Pierpaoli, Walter, M.D., Ph.D.
Regelson, William, M.D.
Colman, Carol
MELATONIN MIRACLE
New York: Simon & Schuster, 1995

Cousins, Norman
ANATOMY OF AN ILLNESS
Pennsylvania: W.W. Norton & Co., 1979

Padus, Emrika
EMOTIONS AND YOUR HEALTH
Pennsylvania: Rodale Press, 1992

Brendan O'Regan
Caryle Hirshberg
SPONTANEOUS REMISSION, An Annotated Bibliography
California, Sausalito: Institute of Noetic Sciences, 1993

Pert, Candace B., Ph.D.
MOLECULES OF EMOTION
New York: Scribner, 1997

Nuland, Sherwin B.
THE WISDOM OF THE BODY
New York: Alfred A. Knopf, Inc., 1997

Hart, Carol
SECRETS OF SEROTONIN
New York: Lynn Sonberg Book Associates, 1996

Braden, Gregg
AWAKENING TO ZERO POINT
Washington: Radio Bookstore Press 1997

Braden, Gregg
WALKING BETWEEN THE WORLDS
Washington: Radio Bookstore Press 1997

Green, Elmer E., Ph.D.
JOURNAL OF TRANSPERSONAL PSYCHOLOGY, Vol. II, No. 1, 1970
Life Sciences Institue
Topeka, Kansas

Norris, Patricia, Ph.D. & Garrett Porter
I CHOOSE LIFE
Stillpoint Publishing
Walpole, New Hamsphire

Every effort has been made to gain permission of previously published material.   Where there has been no reply, I interpret this to mean I am within fair use rights.

POETRY INDEX

ABOUT THE AUTHOR

Life on a farm during the drought and depression of the thirties made survival a common concern. Faith and ingenuity were essential. I attended the University of Nebraska and became a teacher. Later a writing course was completed. Healthful cookbooks were created and published. I was not stymied by a hopeless medical crisis when a religious experience caused improvement. By analyzing the religious feelings, types of healing biofeedback were created. For decades these were useful. Experience enabled me to recognize evolving medical research that could explain such healings. As a mother and grandmother I became dedicated to connecting the pieces.